ATKINS DIET

+

Emotional Eating

Break the Cycle, Say STOP Binge Eating! A Proven 21-Day Program Based on 10 Intuitive Principles for a Healthy Relationship with Food. Loose More Than 125 Pounds

BY
Jessica Davidson

ATKINS DIET

ATKINS DIET

Easier to Follow than Keto, Paleo, Mediterranean or Low-Calorie Diet, Allows You to Lose Weight Quickly, Without Saying Goodbye to Super Prohibited Sweets & Ice Cream in a Diet (Part 1)

BY
Jessica Davidson

Table of Contents

INTRODUCTION 13
CHAPTER 1: HOW DOES ATKINS DIET WORKS? 19
CHAPTER 2: THE BENEFITS OF THE ATKINS DIET 28
CHAPTER 3: THE PHASES OF THE ATKINS DIET FOUR PHASES 43
CHAPTER 4: FOOD LIST OF THE ATKINS DIET 64
CHAPTER 5: BREAKFAST RECIPES 71
    ALMOND AND COCONUT MUFFIN 71
    Almond-Pineapple Smoothie 73
    Atkins Pancakes 74
    Baked Eggs and Asparagus 75
    Atkins Waffles 76

ATKINS DIET

Easier to Follow than Keto, Paleo, Mediterranean or Low-Calorie Diet, Allows You to Lose Weight Quickly, Without Saying Goodbye to Super Prohibited Sweets & Ice Cream in a Diet (Part 2)

BY
Jessica Davidson

Table of Contents

INTRODUCTION 85

CHAPTER 6: HITTING THE DIET BOTTOM 91

Symptoms of Diet Plan Backlash 92
The Paradox of Dieting 95
Dieting Intake Cannot Battle Biology 97
Diet Increases your Risk of Getting More Weight! 100

CHAPTER 7: WHAT TYPE OF EATER ARE YOU? 103

The Eating Personalities 105
When your Eating Personality Works Against You 110
Intuitive Eater Introduction 111
How Your Intuitive Eater Gets Buried 112
Eat Healthy Messages Or Die 113

CHAPTER 8: INTUITIVE EATING STANDARDS: SUMMARY 116

Guideline One: 116
Guideline Two: 117
Guideline Three: 117
Guideline Four: 118
Guideline Five: 119
Guideline Six: 119
Guideline Seven: 121
Guideline Eight: 121
Guideline Nine: 122
Guideline Ten: 123
AN ACTIVITY WITH GREAT REWARDS 123

CHAPTER 9: AROUSING THE INTUITIVE EATER: STAGES 125

Stage One: Readiness-Hitting Diet Plan Bottom 129
Stage Two: Exploration-Conscious Learning And Quest For Pleasure 130

Stage Three: Crystallization 133
Stage 4: The Intuitive Eater Awakens 135
Stage Five: The Ultimate Stage-Treasure The Pleasure 136
That you can do it! 137
CONCLUSION.. 138

EMOTIONAL EATING

Break the Cycle, Say STOP Binge Eating! A Proven 21-Day Program Based on Ten Intuitive Principles for a Healthy Relationship with Food. Be Free from the Slavery of Hunger (Part 1)

By
Kelly Francis

TABLE OF CONTENTS

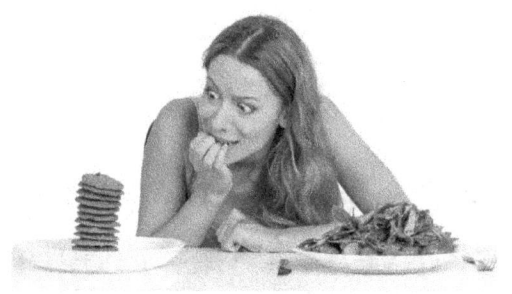

INTRODUCTION 143
CHAPTER 1: COMMON CAUSES OF EMOTIONAL FEEDING 157
CHAPTER 2: ALTERNATIVES TO EMOTIONAL FEEDING 163
CHAPTER 3: DOING THIS STUFF PROVIDES YOUR MIND TIME TO CATCH UP TO YOUR ABDOMEN 178
CHAPTER 4: HOW DOES ONE GO BACK TO ON TRACK?. 183
CHAPTER 5: CONTRIBUTING FACTORS 195

EMOTIONAL EATING

Break the Cycle, Say STOP Binge Eating! A Proven 21-Day Program Based on Ten Intuitive Principles for a Healthy Relationship with Food. Be Free from the Slavery of Hunger (Part 2)

By
Kelly Francis

TABLE OF CONTENTS

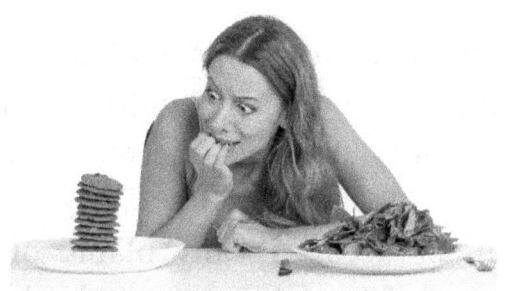

CHAPTER 6: A SIMPLE LIST OF HEALTHY LIVING ACTIVITIES.................... 225

CHAPTER 7: FOODS THAT INVARIABLY PRICE BUT FORTY CENTS PER SERVING................259

CHAPTER 8: TINY HEALTHY HABITS................... 269

CHAPTER 9: FOOD................321

CHAPTER 10: TAKE CHARGE OF YOUR FOOD SETTING..365

CONCLUSION................... 371

© Copyright 2020 - All rights reserved.

The content contained within this book may not be reproduced, duplicated or transmitted without direct written permission from the author or the publisher.

Under no circumstances will any blame or legal responsibility be held against the publisher, or author, for any damages, reparation, or monetary loss due to the information contained within this book. Either directly or indirectly.

Legal Notice:

This book is copyright protected. This book is only for personal use. You cannot amend, distribute, sell, use, quote or paraphrase any part, or the content within this book, without the consent of the author or publisher.

Disclaimer Notice:

Please note the information contained within this document is for educational and entertainment purposes only. All effort has been executed to present accurate, up to date, and reliable, complete information. No warranties of any kind are declared or implied. Readers acknowledge that the author is not engaging in the rendering of legal, financial, medical or professional advice. The content within this book has been derived from various sources. Please consult a licensed professional before attempting any techniques outlined in this book.

By reading this document, the reader agrees that under no circumstances is the author responsible for any losses, direct or indirect, which are incurred as a result of the use of information contained within this document, including, but not limited to, — errors, omissions, or inaccuracies.

Introduction

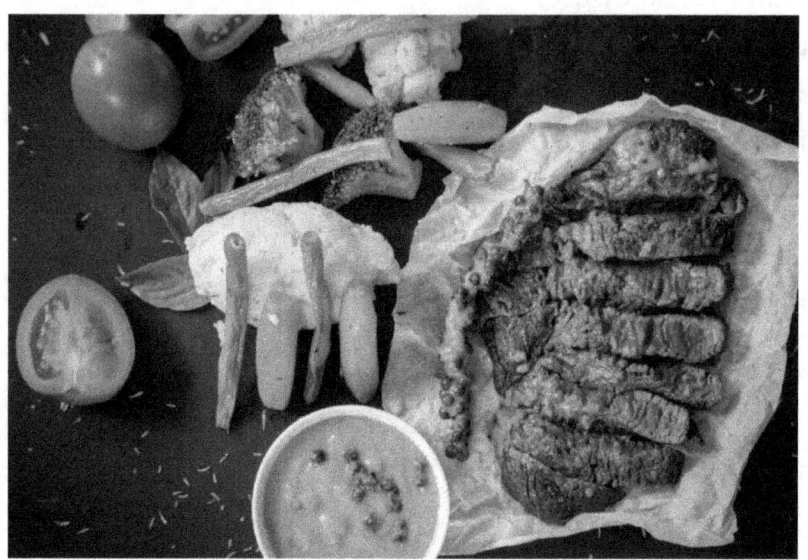

An Introduction to ATKINS Diet
What is Atkins Diet?

The Atkins Diet was created by Dr. Robert Atkins, a cardiologist whose interest in the health benefits of low-carb diets first culminated in the 1972 book "Dr. Atkins Diet Revolution," The diet involves four phases, starting with very few carbs and eating progressively more until you get to your desired weight.

In phase one, for example, you're allowed 20 grams a day of "net carbs," 12 to 15 of them from "foundation vegetables" high in fiber like arugula, cherry tomatoes and Brussels sprouts, according to the traditional Atkins 20 plan. This is advised for maximum weight loss. Two other iterations of the diet, Atkins 40, which the company says is "perfect for those who have less than 40 pounds to lose," and Atkins 100, a plan promoted to those seeking to maintaining their current weight, have a starting point of 40 grams and 100 grams of net carbs per day, respectively.

Generally speaking, the theory is that by limiting carbs, your body has to turn to an alternative fuel – stored fat. So sugars and "simple starches" like potatoes, white bread and rice are all but squeezed out; protein and fat like chicken, meat and eggs are embraced. Fat is burned; pounds come off.

But reducing total carbs isn't all there is to Atkins. Limiting the carbs you take in at any one time is also in the game plan. A carb-heavy meal floods the blood with glucose, too much for the cells to use or to store in the liver as glycogen. Where does it end up? As fat.

In terms of plan flexibility, Atkins 100 allows you to eat the widest variety of foods in the beginning, allocating 100 net carbs throughout the day. Here's how it breaks down:

- A minimum of 12 to 15 grams of net carbs a day of foundation vegetables
- Three 4- to 6-ounce servings of protein a day
- Two to four servings of added fat a day

The remaining 85 grams of net carbs come from foods like legumes, nuts or seeds, higher-carb fruits and vegetables and whole grains.

Low-Carb Diet

These diets provide fewer carbs than is recommended by government guidelines and are known to bring on quick weight loss.

How much does Atkins Diet cost?

Meat and fresh veggies are pricier than most processed and fast foods, so the Atkins Diet is typically more expensive than the average American's. How much more than usual you'll spend will depend largely on your choices of protein sources. Are you buying mostly ground beef or springing for veal? Chicken or turkey? Chuck vs. New York strip? Buying in season should keep the veggie tab reasonable.

Will Atkins Diet help you lose weight?

Atkins and other low-carb diets have been studied longer and harder than most other approaches, and Atkins does appear to be moderately successful, especially in the first couple of weeks. That's only part of the story, however.

Much of the initial loss is water, say experts, because of the diet's diuretic effect. That's true of many other diets, too, and is one of the reasons researchers don't judge diets based on a few weeks of results. In diet studies, long-term generally starts at two years. Here's what several key studies had to say about Atkins and other low-carb diets:

Over short periods, Atkins results vary. In one study, published in 2006 in the British Medical Journal, Atkins dieters lost an average of 10 pounds in the first four weeks while those on meal-replacement (Slim Fast), caloric-restriction (Weight Watchers) and low-fat (Rosemary Conley's "Eat Yourself Slim" book) diets lost 6 to 7 pounds. At the one-month point and thereafter, however, there were no significant differences in weight loss among the groups.

A 2007 study that appeared in the Journal of the American Medical Association divided roughly 300 overweight or obese women into groups and assigned them to one of four types of diets: low-carb (Atkins), low-fat (Ornish), low saturated-fat/moderate-carb (LEARN), and roughly equal parts protein, fat, and carb (Zone). At two months, the Atkins dieters had lost an average of about 9½ pounds compared with 5 to 6 pounds for those on the other three diets. At six months, weight loss for the Atkins group averaged about 13 pounds; the other three groups averaged 4 1/2 to 7 pounds. At 12 months, the Atkins group had lost what researchers called a "modest" 10 pounds; the other dieters averaged 3 1/2 to 6 pounds. Drawing firm conclusions from this study is risky, however. The dropout rate in all four groups was significant, and many participants didn't follow their assigned diet. The Atkins dieters, for example, took in far more carbs than they were supposed to.

A third study, published in 2010 in the Annals of Internal Medicine, found no clear advantage either to a low-carb diet based on Atkins or a generic low-fat diet. Both helped participants lose an average of 11% of their starting weight at 12 months, but they gained about a third of it back after that. At two years, average loss for both diets was 7% of initial body weight. (That's still not bad – if you're overweight, losing just 5 to 10% of your current weight can help stave off some diseases.) An analysis of five studies that compared low-carb and low-fat diets published in 2006 in the Archives of Internal Medicine concluded similarly – while weight loss was greater at six months for low-carb dieters, by 12 months that difference wasn't significant.

It is still unclear, regardless of claims made for low-carb diets, whether the main reason for weight loss is carb restriction specifically or simply cutting calories. A study published in 2009 in the New England Journal of Medicine found that after two years, participants assigned either to a 35% or a 65% carb diet lost about the same amount of weight – 6 to 7 1/2 pounds on average. In 2003, researchers who analyzed about 100 low-carb studies concluded in the Journal of the American Medical Association that weight loss on those diets was associated mostly with cutting calories and not with cutting carbs.

Researchers reviewed 17 different studies that followed a total of 1,141 obese patients on low-carb eating plans, some similar to the Atkins diet. Results were published in 2012 in Obesity. The study shows that low-carb dieters lost an average of nearly 18 pounds over a period of six months to a year. They also saw improvements in their waist circumference.

In a study published in November 2014 in Circulation: Cardiovascular Quality and Outcomes, researchers analyzed existing research on Atkins, South Beach, Weight Watchers and the Zone diets to find out which was most effective. Their findings suggested that none of the four diet plans led to significant weight loss, and none was starkly better than the others when it came to keeping weight off for a year or more. Each of the four plans helped dieters shed about the same number of pounds in the short term: around 5% of their starting body weight. After two years, however, some of the lost weight was regained by those on the Atkins or Weight Watchers plans. Since the diets produce similar results, the study authors concluded that dieters should choose the one that best adheres to their lifestyle – for example, Weight Watchers involved a group-based, behavior-modification approach, and Atkins focuses on lowering carbs.

Following the Atkins Diet will likely seriously challenge your willpower. How much do you love sweet and starchy foods? Would you miss crusty French bread? Pasta? Grape jelly? Diets that severely limit entire food groups for months and years tend to have lower success rates than less-restrictive diets do, and the Atkins Diet is the definition of a restrictive diet.

One study showed higher percentages of Atkins dieters dropping out at three, six, 12 and 24 months than others did on a low-fat diet, but the differences were not significant. Two other studies that included low-carb dieters concluded diet type wasn't connected to dropout rate.

The Atkins Diet isn't known for its convenience. At home, building variety into meals is a little harder than usual. Eating out takes more effort. Alcohol is limited. Company products and online resources may be helpful. In 2013, Atkins launched a frozen-food line, which the company says is the first low-carb frozen-food line on the market.

Atkins recipes abound. Atkins provides meal plans, recipes with ingredient lists and food carb counts, all in print-friendly format. There is at least a smattering of recipes across a range of cuisines from American to Middle Eastern to French to Asian.

Eating out is doable on the Atkins Diet. Just make sure you've read Atkins' list of approved fast-food and cuisine-specific options before heading out (and don't be bashful about asking lots of questions about meal preparation).

Chapter 1: How Does Atkins Diet Works?

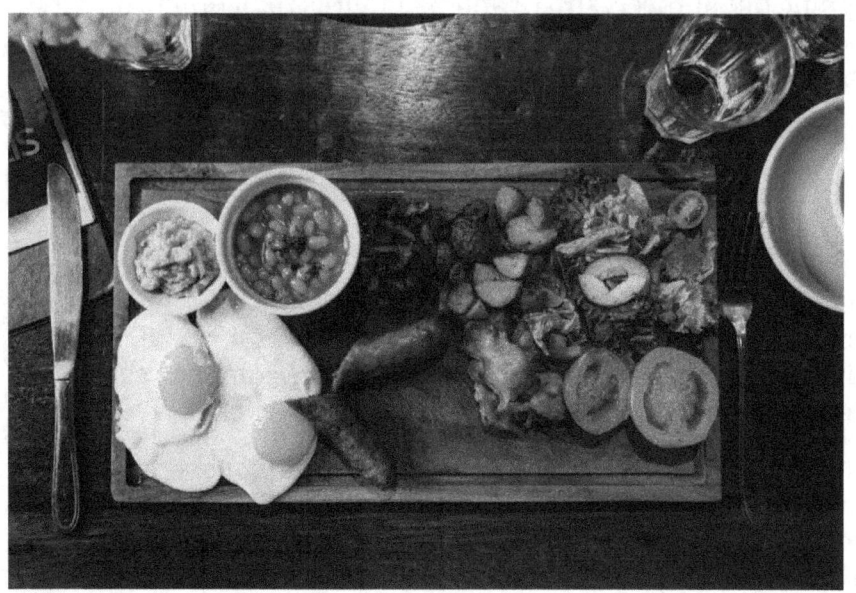

How It Works

The Atkins diet plan relies on knowing how much carbohydrate is in everything you eat. Specifically, consumers count their net carbs. Net carbs can be calculated by checking the total grams of carbohydrate in your portion of food and subtracting the grams of fiber and sugar alcohols or glycerin (if applicable).

There are three Atkins programs based on different levels of net carb intake per day. The company recommends that you check with your healthcare provider for personalized advice before choosing a program to manage a medical condition.

Atkins 20

The Atkins 20 plan is what most would consider to be the classic Atkins plan. It is designed for those who have over 40 pounds to lose, have a waist size of over 35 (for women) or 40 (for men), are pre-diabetic, or diabetic.

People on this program start by consuming just 20 net carbs per day. They eat a variety of approved (foundational) vegetables, lean meat, cheese, and healthy fats to meet their energy needs. After two weeks on Atkins 20, people on this plan can begin to add berries, nuts, and other fiber-rich carb sources in five net carb increments. Then gradually they learn to incorporate healthier carbohydrate choices to reach and maintain their goal weight.

There are four phases to the Atkins 20 program:

Induction Phase. For two weeks or longer, consumers keep their net carbs at the lowest level.

Balancing Phase. People on the program slowly add grams of net carbs to find the best carbohydrate balance.

Fine Tuning Phase. Clients are advised make small tweaks to reach and maintain their goal weight for at least a month.

Lifetime Maintenance. You continue to eat a healthy diet with limited carbohydrates to maintain your goal weight.

Atkins 40

This plan offers a more relaxed program where dieters eat from all food groups from day one. The plan is designed for people who have 40 pounds or less to lose, those who prefer a wider variety of food choices, or for women who are breastfeeding with a goal to lose weight. On this program, you start the first phase of the plan by consuming 40 grams of net carbs per day from vegetables, fruits, nuts, legumes, and whole grains. As dieters approach their goal weight, they add carbs in 10 net carb increments to find their personal carb "sweet spot" to maintain their healthy weight.

Atkins 100

This is the most relaxed Atkins eating program. It is designed for those who want to maintain their current weight, who prefer the widest variety of food choices, or for women who are breastfeeding and have a goal to maintain weight. The company also suggests this program for women who are pregnant as long as they have approval from their healthcare provider. On this plan, you consume about 100 grams of net carb per day with no foods that are off limits.

On each of the Atkins plans, net carbs are to be divided between three meals and two snacks per day so that blood sugar remains stable throughout the day. You don't count calories on these programs, but portion size recommendations are provided. Additionally, it recommended that certain foods (such as added fats) are limited.

Pros and Cons

Consumers who choose to go on an Atkins eating plan are likely to see some weight loss and health benefits.

For many people, restricting carbohydrates means eliminating heavily processed, high-sugar, high-starch foods which contribute calories without substantial nutrition.

If you replace those less healthy foods with more nutritious foods (such as those on the Atkins Acceptable Foods lists), you are likely to increase your intake of important micro and macronutrients.

On the flip side, however, if you currently consume a standard American diet, adjusting to an Atkins plan may be challenging, especially if you choose to go on the Atkins 20 plan. Typically, people consume most of their calories from carbohydrate. Cutting back on carbs can lead to symptoms including headaches, fatigue, mood swings, and constipation.

Additionally, even though you don't have to count calories on the Atkins diet, you do need to count carbs, calculate net carbs and balance carbs between meals and snacks. You'll also need to use food lists to make sure you're consuming foods that are compliant. For many busy people, this work may seem overwhelming. As an alternative, consumers can choose to purchase an Atkins meal plan and get pre-packaged meals, smoothies, and snacks.

Pros

If you are interested in the Atkins diet, there are substantial studies documenting the benefits of going on the low-carb diet. Many of these published studies have supported the use of the program for weight loss and other health benefits.

Weight Loss

The Atkins diet has a long history of successful weight loss. Many people have lost weight on this plan and the program has been studied in numerous clinical trials. But if you are considering Atkins for weight loss or weight maintenance, you'll find that there is a range of studies with conflicting results.

A study published in JAMA compared the Atkins diet to LEARN (Lifestyle, Exercise, Attitudes, Relationships, and Nutrition, a program that is low in fat and high in carbohydrate based on national guidelines), Zone, and Ornish diets in overweight pre-menopausal women. Researchers found that those following Atkins lost more weight and experienced more favorable overall metabolic effects at 12 months.

Another analysis of studies published in the journal Nutrients compared Atkins to 19 other diets without specific calories targets. The researchers determined that of the diets evaluated, the Atkins diet showed the most evidence in producing clinically meaningful short-term and long-term weight loss.

However, there is also substantial research comparing high fat ketogenic diets (such as Atkins) to diets where calories are restricted. Several of these studies have shown that there is no difference between caloric restriction and carb restriction for long-term weight loss. Additionally, while there is some support for low-carb, higher fat diets, there are still medical experts who question whether or not the diet is healthy or effective for the long-term.

Results from a large nutritional study were reported in 2019 at both the American Society of Nutrition and the American Diabetes Association conferences. The findings suggest that there isn't necessarily a single diet that meets the needs of every person trying to lose weight because each body responds differently. These findings support research published in other scientific journals suggesting that the best diet for weight loss is the diet you can stick to for the long-term.

Some studies have demonstrated that Atkins and other ketogenic diets are effective for weight loss. However, other studies have concluded that cutting carbs is no more effective than cutting calories, especially over the long-term. This has led many researchers to suggest that the best eating and lifestyle program for weight loss and weight maintenance is the plan you can stick to for life.

No Calorie Counting

There is growing frustration over the use of calorie counting for weight loss and weight maintenance. Even though most nutrition experts acknowledge the importance of consuming the right number of calories each day, they acknowledge that trying to track and monitor your intake every day can be tedious and may feel restrictive.

On the Atkins plan, you watch your net carb intake but there is no need to count or restrict calories. For many people, this feature of the Atkins plan is most appealing.

Hearty Eating Plan

Some people like the fact that you can eat more rich and satisfying food on the Atkins diet plan. For example, some people prefer this diet because hearty foods like steaks and burgers can stay on their menu.

Protein-rich foods and foods with more fat tend to be satiating. When you feel satisfied after eating, you're likely to delay your next meal or snack and may consume fewer calories overall as a result. In fact, some studies have shown that total caloric intake is lower on the Atkins plan than on other plans with higher carbohydrate intake.

It is important to note, however, that the most current versions of Atkins provide recommendations for portion size. For example, during Phase 1, the recommended daily intake for added fat is just 2-4 tablespoons. So you can't expect to be successful on the Atkins plan if you eat large portions of fatty meat, butter, and cheese.

Clearly Defined Guidelines

Those who prefer a structured approach to eating will enjoy Atkins. Each phase of the program has a specific time or weight goal that is clearly explained.

For example, Phase 1 lasts for two weeks (in most situations). Phase 2 lasts until you are 10 pounds from your goal weight. Phase 3 lasts until have been comfortably at your goal weight for four weeks. Extensive lists of acceptable foods are available for each stage and portion sizes for each food category are clearly defined.

Focus on Healthy Carbs

The Atkins diet eliminates refined carbohydrates such as baked goods (like cake and white bread) and encourages the intake of healthy carbohydrates (such as green vegetables and fiber-rich berries), especially in the later stages of the plan. So you learn the difference between good carbs and bad carbs.

For many people, simply reducing the intake of refined grains and sugary foods provides noticeable benefits right away. Drinking water instead of soda and replacing starchy side dishes with foundation vegetables is likely to help you have steady energy levels throughout the day. In addition, you'll lose water weight almost immediately if you cut back on your carb intake.

Resources Widely Available

You'll find most of what you need to follow the Atkins plan online. Food lists and other guides are provided on their website. You'll also find Atkins books and guides in bookstores and online.

If you don't like to prepare your own food all the time, Atkins snack bars and other meal replacements are conveniently available in many markets and discount stores.

Cons

While some dieters enjoy the diet's benefits, others struggle to stick to Atkins' strict eating plan.

Reduced Fruit and Grain Intake

If you're a person who loves fruit, you might struggle on the Atkins plan. Even if you don't love fruit, the USDA recommends that you consume about two cups per day to get the important vitamins and nutrients that they provide.

Eventually, you can add some fruit but in the early stages of the diet, you'll need to avoid healthy foods like berries, bananas, apple, and citrus fruits in order to get into ketosis. Once you are closer to your goal weight, you may be able to consume small amounts of low-carb fruits (such as raspberries) but some people aren't able to stay in ketosis when they consume any fruit.

Grain intake is another concern on the Atkins diet. On the Atkins diet grain-based foods are restricted—especially in the early phases.

Chapter 2: The Benefits Of The Atkins Diet

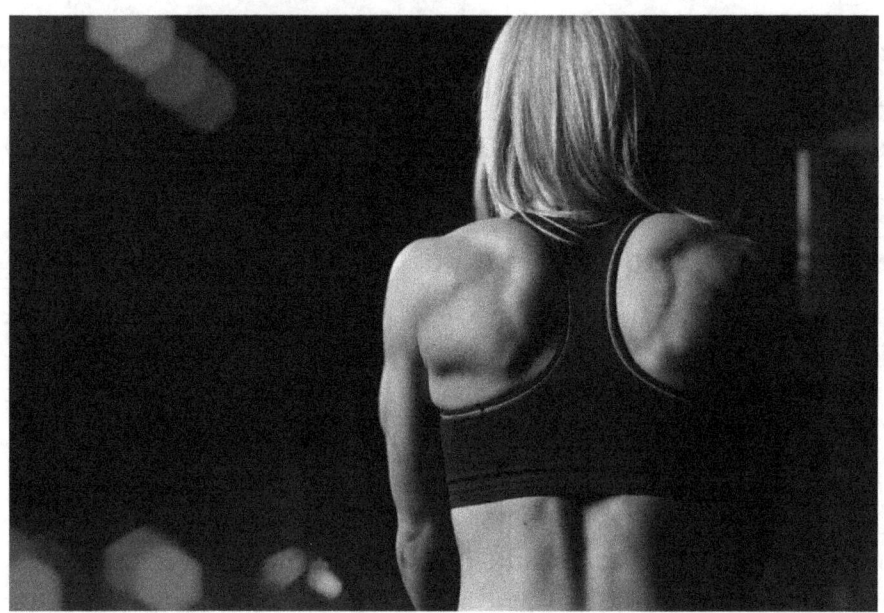

15 Health Benefits of the Atkins Diet

What are the health benefits of the Atkins diet?

This diet is usually recommended for people who are looking for a fairly quick way to achieve weight loss goals, but eating a low-carb diet will provide individuals with a wide range of valuable health benefits.

There have been more than 20 different studies to look at how this diet impacts weight loss and leads to other health improvements, and the diet has become a popular option around the world for people seeking enhanced wellness – without the stress of constantly monitoring your calorie intake.

One: The Atkins diet will improve your heart health.

Researchers who examined 17 different studies of overweight people found that following a low-carb, high-fat diet had a 98 per cent greater chance of lowering the risk of stroke or heart attack than a low-fat diet. Because of how carbohydrates trigger your body to rapidly produce insulin, you'll also end up holding onto excess fat for your body to use as fuel later, when your blood sugar crashes.

Cutting your intake of carbohydrates had a direct impact on your heart health several ways – decreasing your level of triglycerides, raising your levels of "good" cholesterol's, lowering your "bad" cholesterols, and even helping to reduce blood pressure.

Two: The Atkins diet will help you lose weight.

Some followers of the Atkins diet have managed to lose more than 100 pounds – but your individual weight loss results will depend heavily on your adherence to the plan. Since a low-carb diet helps stimulate your body to burn fat, and a diet high in protein and fat helps suppress your appetite, it's easy to see how the Atkins diet can lead to significant weight loss. However, you will need to pay close attention to the carbohydrate counts in everything you eat, as it can add up quickly and impede your potential weight loss results.

You'll see even better results if you mix in a bit of exercise. With the additional energy you'll have from eating clean and enjoying a strong metabolism, shoot for about 150 minutes each week of moderate-intensity exercise.

Three: The Atkins diet will improve blood sugar levels.

Uncontrolled sugar levels are a major risk factor for both heart disease and obesity – and the Atkins diet, particularly during the induction phase, can drastically improve your body's ability to properly process sugar. Even patients taking insulin before embarking on an Atkins diet were able to stop using insulin after changing their nutritional approach.

Limiting your intake of carbohydrates also helps to prevent blood sugar spikes, which are generally triggered by the glycemic content of high-carbohydrate foods. A low-glycemic diet is an effective way of dealing with that, but a low-glycemic diet combined with a reduced intake of carbohydrates is even better.

Four: The Atkins diet can prevent metabolic syndrome.

Most of the symptoms and risk factors that combine into what we know as metabolic syndrome can be treated with the nutritional approach of the Atkins diet. Abdominal obesity, elevated cholesterol, diabetes, and hypertension can all be addressed through this dietary strategy, and thanks to the healthy intake of protein, you can ensure that your muscle mass is preserved.

Maintaining muscle mass helps you keep your body's metabolism running efficiently, allowing you to continue burning fat and improving your overall wellness.

Five: The Atkins diet can help control your appetite.

You'll probably suffer through some cravings at first, especially during the induction phase as you try to cut out carbs almost entirely – but by eliminating the constant spikes and drops in your blood sugar, you'll enjoy a suppressed appetite. Not only will your Atkins diet help eliminate your cravings, you'll also be eating healthier meals more frequently, keeping you well-satiated.

If you do find yourself struggling with cravings, break up your meals with healthy snacks, drink more water, and make sure there isn't an emotional reason behind your physical food cravings. Once you get more familiar with your body, you'll be able to tell what's triggering your cravings and deal with them appropriately.

Six: The Atkins diet will boost brain function.

Low-carb diets have a reputation for negatively affecting your brain function, since your brain needs carbs for energy. However, once followers have gotten past the initial phase of reducing carbohydrate intake and their bodies have had a chance to adjust to a new metabolic process, the increased consumption of brain-healthy fats and B-complex vitamins found in leafy green vegetables work to produce more brain hormones like serotonin.

Low-carb fruits like berries also help enhance communication networks between your brain cells, promoting brain cell survival and regeneration.

Seven: The Atkins diet can provide increased physical endurance.

While scientists have long known how the Atkins diet can increase weight loss and the body's ability to effectively and efficiently burn fat, studies are now being done to examine how the diet could augment the body's physical performance and recovery.

According to some research, these athletes proved to be "very healthy," even "beyond what you can achieve with good genetics and extensive training," said Jeff Volek, lead researcher and professor of human sciences at the Ohio State University. Volek added that the restriction of carbs allows the body's fat-burning program to "reboot" and enable athletes to reach significantly improved levels of performance and health.

Eight: The Atkins diet can help clear your skin.

Studies have shown that the Atkins diet has a positive effect on a variety of chronic and unpleasant skin conditions – clearing up some of the redness, itching, and irritation associated with psoriasis, eczema, acne, and even vitiligo. Not only that, but even in practitioners without ongoing skin concerns, eating a low-carb diet can make your skin feel and look more radiant, moisturized, and healthy.

These benefits also impact your hair and your nails, which will all be stronger and healthier. The increased intake of vitamins and minerals you'll get from eating more vegetables and fruits will have a major effect how you feel inside and outside.

Nine: The Atkins diet will help you eat more nutrients.

By focusing your diet on whole, unprocessed foods, you'll enjoy eating far greater quantities of nutrients like vitamins, minerals, and antioxidants – all of which will directly impact your health and well-being. These nutrient-dense foods have a number of varied properties that will all provide a range of health benefits, which you wouldn't get if you were eating a plate of spaghetti or a pizza instead.

Your meals should include an adequate portion of protein along with an array of high-fiber, low-glycemic fruits and vegetables. This encourages you to eat different kinds of produce and get different kinds of nutrients, achieving a well-balanced, healthy diet.

Ten: The Atkins diet will decrease inflammation.

Inflammation is an important part of your body's defense system, and a certain amount is to be expected in any healthy individual – especially during times of illness or injury. However, chronic inflammation can lead to serious health concerns like cancer, heart disease, and even neurological disorders like Alzheimer's and Parkinson's.

A lot of this inflammation can be attributed to the insulin spikes that come from eating processed foods and sugars, including carbs. Eating a variety of foods that decrease inflammation, like those recommended on the Atkins diet, can prevent chronic inflammation from causing lasting damage.

Eleven: The Atkins diet will improve digestion.

While your digestive system will likely need a bit of time to adjust to your new eating habits, a low-carb diet has proven to improve overall digestion. Thanks to the increased fiber intake found within the Atkins diet, you'll enjoy a heathy digestive system and reduced acid reflux, heartburn, and bloating.

Initially, you may find you are more flatulent than usual, but as your body gets used to your nutritional intake, you'll find that you suffer from gas less, as well.

Twelve: The Atkins diet can help prevent cancer.

A nutrition plan that focuses on getting enough healthy fats can drastically reduce your chances of developing certain types of cancers. Cancer growth happens when your body is running inefficiently, creating a breeding ground for developing infections. Uncontrolled blood sugar is a major trigger for this development, but the Atkins diet has proven effective at keeping these levels stable.

The reduced inflammation also helps keep your body's immune response functioning effectively, and helps your body react effectively to stress.

Thirteen: The Atkins diet targets abdominal fat deposits.

Excess fat that has accumulated around your midsection can lead to a number of health risks – impacting almost every organ in your body by producing excess chemicals and hormones. Major concerns include type 2 diabetes, colorectal cancer, and cardiovascular disease.

This fat is troublesome to lose and easy to put on, but can be reduced thanks to three major factors – exercise, sleep, and diet. The Atkins diet gives you the tools to tackle all three, starting with your nutritional intake.

Fourteen: The Atkins diet can enhance sleep quality.

With your increased consumption of nutrients, healthy amounts of fat and protein, and stable blood sugar, your body will be under less stress and feeling much healthier and more energetic. This will dramatically reduce the time you spend fighting insomnia, meaning you'll be able to fall asleep faster and stay asleep longer.

The quality of your rest will also be improved thanks to the brain-boosting power of the Atkins diet, and the added energy you'll see from all the nutrients you're putting in your body.

Fifteen: The Atkins diet helps with weight maintenance.

Once you've reached the fourth phase of the Atkins diet, you'll be in maintenance mode. With most diets, followers use this as an opportunity to return to their regular eating habits – and will end up piling all that lost weight right back on.

However, since Atkins is considered a life-long nutritional approach instead of a temporary diet, you'll have much better luck maintaining your weight loss and health benefits. Introduce carbohydrates slowly, and if you start having cravings, lower your intake. Switching between the third and fourth phases while keeping an eye on your overall health is a great way to keep those pounds off and enjoy the healthy lifestyle Atkins delivers.

What should I keep in mind when starting this diet?

If these great health benefits have convinced you to cut down on your carbohydrate intake and begin eating an Atkins-inspired diet, there are some things you should keep in mind as you set out on your new journey. While the benefits of the Atkins diet far outweigh any of the challenges that come along with it, it's important to know what obstacles you might come across – especially during your first few weeks on the diet.

Fortunately, you'll feel so good on this diet that you'll have no trouble overlooking these minor issues. It's easy to make a change when you know how huge the payoff is – and the Atkins diet is a great step along the way to lasting health and wellness.

Carb crash is a real thing.

When you're used to eating plenty of carbohydrates, it's normal and even expected to feel a bit of discomfort during the first few days of cutting back. You might find yourself missing these foods and craving them with a startling intensity, but there are some ways you can distract yourself enough to move past this initial phase of withdrawal.

- **Get plenty of fiber and fat.** Together, these foods can provide your body with some much-needed satiety. Flax seeds are a great option to get both of these at once, or salads with a lean protein added.

- **Snack frequently.** Don't go more than three hours without eating a healthy, low-carb snack, especially during your withdrawal from carbs. If you can avoid being hungry, you'll have better luck fighting cravings.

- **Find things you want to eat.** This diet is strict, but there are still tons of delicious things you can eat on an Atkins diet. Discover approved foods that you'll look forward to eating so your body will begin to crave those healthy alternatives, instead of carbohydrates.

- **Do something for yourself.** You're making a great change to improve your well-being, so instead of indulging in an unhealthy craving, do something else you enjoy. Read a book, take a bubble bath, or turn to a loved one for some support and encouragement.

Even once you're out of that initial withdrawal phase, some people experience a second period of "carb crash" where they have reported symptoms of feeling "off." Some people feel jittery or shaky, some feel fatigued, and some feel irritable. These symptoms will disappear after a couple of days, but you can try to prevent them from being overwhelming by indulging in a serving of low-carb fruit.

This can also be caused by a lack of salt, since many people on the Atkins diet will lose quite a bit of water weight within the first few days – which means a loss of sodium. If low-carb fruit doesn't help relieve the symptoms, try drinking a cup of bouillon a few times a day – and ensure that you are getting plenty of potassium.

You're going to have to learn to count carbs.

This sounds a lot more intimidating than it is, but there is definitely a learning curve involved with carb counting. The more you do it, the easier it will get – but in the beginning, a trip to the grocery store will be a little more involved than you're probably used to.

Since the induction phase of the Atkins diet has a strict requirement of under 20 grams of carbs each day, you will need to read food labels carefully to make sure you stay under your carb limit. Once you've passed this stage, you will be able to add more low-carb foods to your diet, and eventually reach a point where you can consume as many healthy carbs as your body can handle without gaining weight – but you'll always need to be thinking about what's in the foods you're eating.

When reading product labels, be sure to check the serving size as well as the carbohydrate count. If you are going to be eating more of a specific food, you may need to double or triple the total carbohydrate number in order to get an accurate estimate of what your intake will be.

Some people find it easier to count carbs by tracking each meal on an app that gives a breakdown of the nutritional content of your daily food intake. This way, you'll be able to clearly see how much carbohydrate is in the foods you eat, and then you can make the necessary adjustments to stay within the recommended range.

Eating an Atkins diet is time consuming.

If you're the kind of person who usually grabs food on the go, you'll have to make some big changes in order to adjust to an Atkins-style diet. It's hard to find readily available foods that will fit the restrictions of this diet, so be prepared to either make most of your meals yourself, or ask for modified versions of foods on most restaurant menus.

Even grocery shopping will take longer initially, as you learn about carbohydrates and calculate how much of each food you'll be able to eat. This will get easier with time, though, and soon you'll be able to hit the store and get what you need without a second thought.

You'll also be spending more time in the kitchen, prepping meals and cooking for yourself or for your family. If you have more free time on the weekends, you can always do the prep work in advance and come home to heat up pre-portioned servings of Atkins-approved meals. This is a great way to teach yourself to cook and learn your way around the kitchen, though, and like carb counting, it will get easier with practice.

This diet is a lifestyle change.

Eating an Atkins diet isn't just about losing weight – it's about making valuable changes to your entire lifestyle to achieve long-term health benefits. Sure, you'll probably see fat loss and watch the number on the scale go down, but in order to maintain these results, you'll need to look at Atkins as a lifestyle commitment.

Surrounding yourself with supportive people is a great way to ensure you can stick to this diet and make it a life-long habit. It might be difficult at first, to go out for dinner and drinks with friends and stick to Atkins-approved choices, but if you're with people who want to see you succeed, you'll be able to keep your social commitments while sticking to your Atkins diet.

Also, you might want to pack healthy, approved snacks for instances where other people are snacking around you – like when someone brings donuts or chips to the office, or at a party with tons of processed junk foods. If you have something quick and easy on-hand to snack on instead of indulging in the foods you've worked hard to avoid, you won't be nearly as tempted to cheat on your healthy new lifestyle.

How can I get started?

If you normally eat a diet that includes a variety of carbohydrates, making the switch to a diet like Atkins can be pretty intimidating. A good rule to keep in mind is to stick to unprocessed, natural, whole foods as much as you can. This will help you limit your intake of foods that aren't included on your diet plan without having to spend too much time thinking about it.

Take the list of approved Atkins foods to the grocery store and pick up everything you need to get started with these low-carb meal options. These recipes will help you get started on your journey to Atkins-style eating, helping you lose weight and achieve a wide range of important health benefits. Keep in mind that most of your shopping should happen along the outside edges of the store – most of the aisles are full of processed foods.

As you practice making these Atkins-friendly meals, you'll learn more about low-carb eating and start coming up with your own inspired recipes. Hopefully your journey to healthier eating will help you discover new foods you didn't even know you liked, and motivate you to maintain your beneficial Atkins lifestyle.

Chapter 3: The Phases Of The Atkins Diet Four Phases

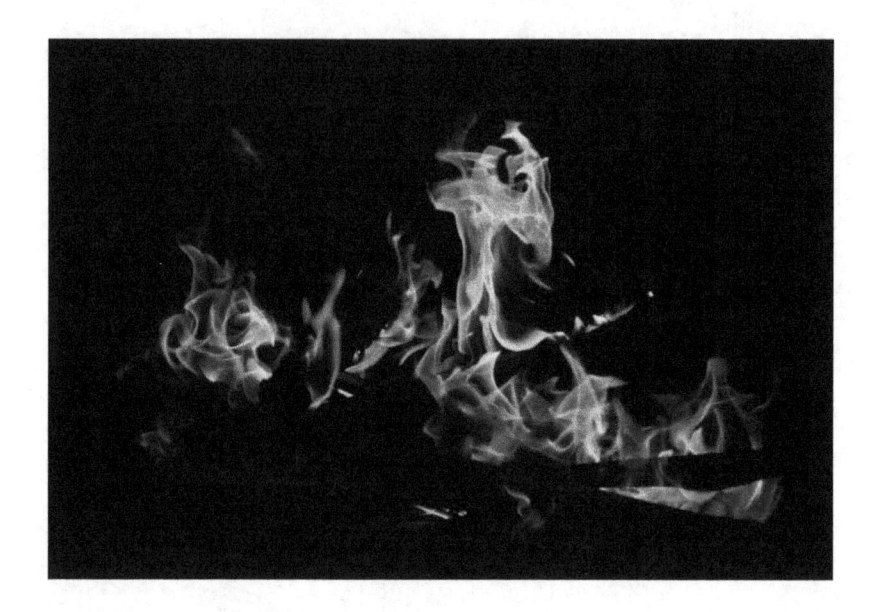

The Atkins diet has four phases:

Phase 1 – Induction

What You Eat On in The Induction Phase

From day one on Induction – you can eat all types of meat, fish, shellfish as well as a huge range of salads and vegetables. You will notice that there are no carbs in meat and fish while the number of net carbs in the vegetables in phase one are quite low. In the Induction phase, 12- 15g of your daily carbs should come from the foundation vegetables listed under phase one.

The next step is to turn lists of food into meals. We found the easiest approach for the first two weeks was to simply follow the meal plans at the back of the New Atkins New You book. Alternatively, the Starter Box comes with a Quick Start Guide with a two-week meal plan. Another option is the meal planner on the Atkins site – it has hundreds of meals to choose from so whatever your preferences and tastes you will be able to put together a meal plan to suit you – check out the Atkins recipes here or click on 'Create your plan' on this page. The foods you get to eat on Atkins from day one really are delicious so prepare to enjoy!

The advantage of following one of the meal plans above is that the carbs are already calculated for each meal and add up to the recommended 20g per day. Feel free to repeat meals you like or substitute other vegetables, side dishes, snacks or desserts as desired as long as the carb counts are comparable. To check how many carbs are in a food just check the Acceptable Food List. You receive a carb counter book in your Starter Box which includes a comprehensive list of foods and their carb counts.

As you get used to counting carbs, it is a good idea to experiment with different recipes to make sure you find meals that will suit your tastes, budget, time constraints etc. After all, you will not stick to this way of eating if you don't like the food so it's worth putting in the effort to make sure you do customize it to your tastes and lifestyle. The New Atkins New You book has lots of tips to help everyone to follow this program no matter what your culinary preferences, whether you eat out a lot or whether you are vegetarian or vegan!

What is off limits?

The part that everyone thinks is going to be the most difficult with the Atkins diet is the idea of giving up bread, baked products and foods like pasta. You probably won't believe this now but once you stop eating high carb foods like this, you also stop craving them! So for Paul and I, passing up on a slice of toast or a scone is no act of willpower, we simply don't want them anymore. And this kicks in very quickly – after two weeks or even less. So for now just take our word for it – it is much easier than you think it will be! Also it really is better if you do not cheat on this because if you do, you will just start the cravings all over again. So here is a list of what is off limits in Induction:

- Caloric fizzy drinks
- Fruits and fruit juices (other than lemon and lime juice and any fruits listed on the Acceptable Food List)
- Foods made with flour or other grain products – bread, cereal, pasta, muffins, scones, biscuits, crisps, cakes and products like gravy and packet mixes which usually contain flour
- Sugar, sweets and any foods containing added sugar – check the carb amounts on the label.
- Junk food in any form.
- Grains – even whole grains, rice, oats, barley etc.
- Alcohol (but don't worry you can re-introduce it in a few weeks' time in Phase 2)
- Any vegetables not on the Acceptable Food List including starchy vegetables like potatoes, carrots and parsnips. Don't worry however – there is a list of more than 50 other vegetables you can eat!
- On Induction you can eat dairy products such as cream, sour cream, butter and the hard cheeses listed on the Acceptable Food List. However other dairy products including milk (especially low-fat or skimmed milk), cottage cheese, ricotta or yoghurt are

off-limits.
- 'Low-fat' foods or 'diet' products – they are usually surprisingly high in carbohydrates so steer clear.
- Any foods with manufactured trans-fats – this may be listed as hydrogenated or partially-hydrogenated oils.

The list above is not a complete list but use your common sense and stick to the Acceptable Food List and you'll be fine. Also if you have any questions, just ask your Atkins Support Partner.

Top Tips for Induction

The top tips for Induction are:

- Take some time to plan your meals for week one. This way of eating may be quite different from what you are used to so give yourself some time to prepare. This way of eating will become second nature in no time but it is going to require some extra time and effort at the beginning.
- Although you will probably find you are eating more vegetables than you did previously, it is recommended that you take a daily multivitamin and an omeaga-3 fatty acid supplement.
- Buy a notebook and write down what you eat and the amount of carbs at least for the first few weeks. We all selectively remember what we did (or didn't eat!) otherwise. Believe me, this step alone will make a big difference.
- Take a photo before you start. Wear something figures hugging and take a side and front profile pic. You will be so glad you did in a few weeks or months' time when you can compare photos from then with the 'before' picture and see your progress. Also take

your measurements – you'll find a measuring tape in your Starter Box. This is important because sometimes you will see the difference in inches before you see it on the scales.

The Starter Box also includes a weight and measurement tracker. The actual number on the scales is not important. You just need to know what it is so you can see what progress you've made in two weeks' time.

- One of the science based changes in the New Atkins is the recommendation to drink 2 cups of broth, half a teaspoon of salt or 2 tablespoons of regular soya sauce. For Irish readers, you might be familiar with Bovril. As with any diet, you will lose a certain amount of water at the beginning. For some, this can be too much of a good thing as it causes you to lose salts as well and for some people this can cause them to feel tired or weak or to have headaches when they start the Atkins diet. Drinking 2 cups of Bovril will prevent these symptoms. And no this does not make Atkins a high sodium diet!
- Don't forget that sugar is off limits so remember to buy sweetener like sucralose (Splenda), saccharine (Sweet'N Low), stevia (Sweet Leaf or Truvia) or xylitol and have that in your tea or coffee instead of sugar (if you take sugar). Have no more than 3 packets a day and count each packet as 1g of carbs. Also a good idea to get one of the little containers to keep in your handbag (or pocket for the men?!). Most cafes will have sweetener however but still handy to have particularly when visiting friends.
- Milk including skimmed milk is naturally rich in milk sugar (lactose) so its off-limits in Induction. However, cream is an acceptable and delicious alternative in tea/coffee! Just buy fresh cream or double cream – it really is lovely – and once you try it

you'll never want to go back!
- Eat 3 meals and 2 snacks every day. Don't skip meals or go more than 6 waking hours without eating. You should definitely not be hungry on this diet!
- Drink lots of water.
- Don't forget to stock up on your Atkins products so you have suitable snacks to hand at all times. Keep them in your desk at work, your car, handbag – that way you always have a healthy low carb option to hand – they are particularly good if you are out-and-about or busy. You can have two products a day and you certainly will not feel deprived when eating snacks like the delicious Chocolate Chip Daybreak bar or the Advantage Chocolate Crunch bar or the like! The shakes are delicious and very convenient as well. As well as tasting good, the bars (especially the Advantage range) are very filling so they will fill you up and stop you for reaching for unsuitable high-carb alternatives.
- Check the amount of carbohydrates on labels of everything you buy – don't assume anything is low in carbs. In Ireland, you can just go by the total amount of carbohydrates on the label (on the Atkins site you may see comments about deducting fiber from the carb amount – this is because the labeling is different in the US and includes fiber in the carbohydrate count). However, you will probably find you are buying much less food that comes with labels with this way of eating in any case i.e. meat, poultry, fish and vegetables.

By starting the Atkins diet, you are embarking on a journey that will make a huge difference to your health and well-being – congratulations for taking that first step! Your Atkins Support Partner is there to help you, so be sure to take advantage of that.

Phase 2 – Ongoing Weight Loss

Phase 2 is also called Ongoing Weight Loss or **OWL**. Most people spend the majority of their weight loss time in this phase. Initially the differences between Induction and OWL are very small. In OWL, the idea is that you gradually reintroduce other carbohydrate foods bit by bit, while continuing to lose weight.

- Gradually add carbohydrates in the form of nutrient-dense foods, increasing to 25 grams of Net Carbs per day the first week, and moving up each week or every several weeks by 5-gram increments until weight loss stops.
- Continue to stay in control of your appetite and lose weight.
- Find your Carbohydrate Level for Losing (CLL) i.e. the amount of carbohydrates you can eat each day and continue to lose weight.

MOVING ON.

It is really important that you do move into OWL and you do not stay in Induction until you have reached your goal weight. The reason for this is so that you find out what foods you can eat, whether there are carbohydrate foods you are intolerant to and get closer to what will be a permanent way of eating so you maintain your goal weight once you reach it. By the end of OWL you will have an individualized eating plan – it is based on what you have discovered during this process works for you and your body. This is all geared towards making sure that once you have lost the extra weight, it stays lost!

The Carb Ladder

The following carb ladder shows you the order in which you re-introduce carbohydrate foods in OWL. You will already be eating the foods from Rung 1 and Rung 2 from Induction (if you started in Induction). You reintroduce the other foods starting with Rung 3 in Phase 2:

Rung 1: Foundation vegetables – leafy greens and other low-carb vegetables

Rung 2: Dairy foods low in carbs – cream, sour cream and most hard cheeses

Rung 3: Nuts and seeds including nut and seed butters.

Rung 4: Berries, cherries and melon (not watermelon).

Rung 5: Whole milk yoghurt and fresh cheeses, such as cottage cheese and ricotta.

Rung 6: Legumes, including chickpeas, lentils, edamame and the like.

Rung 7: Tomato and vegetable juice "cocktail" and more lemon and lime juice.

Rung 8: Other fruits (not fruit juices or dried fruits)

Rung 9: Starchy vegetables such as winter squash, carrots, peas in pods

Rung 10: Whole grains (not refined grain products)

The foods on the lower rungs are the foods you should be eating most often. On the top rungs are foods that will put in an appearance only occasionally, rarely or never depending on your carb tolerance. So as you can see from the carb ladder and the Atkins food pyramid below you will continue to eat a variety of meat, fish & poultry as well as an abundance of vegetables as well as including healthy fats.

Tips for Success

One important point to keep in mind with OWL is that you will be increasing the range of food you eat in OWL but does does not mean you will be increasing the amount by very much. As with Induction, you should definitely not be hungry so let your appetite be your guide.

The best way to do OWL is to introduce one new food from a group at a time. So for instance you might move on to berries and start by eating a small portion of blueberries. Assuming they cause no problems, you could move on to strawberries in a day or two. What you want to look out for and pay attention to is whether the new food reawakens food cravings, causes gastric distress or interferes with your weight loss. If a food does cause any problems, you can just leave it out and try re-introducing it at a later stage.

If you have been estimating carb counts, now is the time to start counting them. We would recommend that you write down what you eat each day along with the carb counts. That way you will know exactly where you are and it will make it easy to identify if there is a particular food that reawakens cravings or interferes with your weight-loss or causes any other health issues. Ordinarily most of us don't pay enough attention to how we feel and what foods might have caused this but this is a great opportunity to do just that and keeping a food diary and introducing foods one by one makes it much easier.

Now that you are in Phase 2 you can eat all of the convenient and delicious Atkins products including the delicious Endulge bars like the Endulge Chocolate Crisp, Endulge Peanut Caramel and the Endulge Coconut bar. Make sure that you have your Advantage or Daybreak bars or shakes on hand when you are out and about so that you don't resort to eating inappropriate high carb foods.

Phase 3 – Pre-Maintenance

By the time you move to Phase 3, you will be close to achieving your goal weight with just 10 pounds to go. You will also have identified foods that your body can or cannot handle as well as the amount of carbohydrates you can eat daily and continue losing weight. You will almost certainly have noticed other health benefits and improvements in general well-being by now as well. Congratulations!

Phase 3 continues this important process of learning exactly what you need to know to make sure the weight stays lost and you maintain the slim new you. So the objectives of the Pre-Maintenance phase are:

Lose the last 10 pounds slowly – it is tempting to want to get to your goal weight as quickly as possible but its important that you do slow it down as you move towards a permanent way of eating. It may take several months to reach your goal weight, losing perhaps just half a pound a week. Those last few pounds and centimeters can be the most stubborn so it is normal for it to slow down at this stage. If you rush to lose those last few pounds you may never learn what you need to know to keep them off for good..

Test your carb tolerance – as you slow down your weight loss you may be able to increase your Carbohydrate Level for Losing (CLL). The CLL was the number you discovered at the end of Phase 2 – the amount of grams of carbs you can eat each day and continue to lose weight. Now that you are slowing down the weight loss and moving to weight maintenance, you may be able to increase this number.

- Test your tolerance for additional foods – as in Phase 2 you can re-introduce whole food carbohydrates

and note how they make you feel. These will be foods at the top of the carbohydrate ladder (see below) like fruit higher in carbs, starchy veg and unprocessed whole grains. It is important to pay attention to how you feel when you introduce new foods. For example, it they cause cravings to come back or any other adverse effects on your health or well-being it's best to eliminate them. And fantastic that you have discovered this – many people go through life eating foods they are intolerant to and suffering the effects of this.
- Find your ACE (Atkins Carbohydrate Equilibrium) – this is the number of grams of carbs you can eat daily and neither gain or lose weight. This is the magic number that will help you stay at your goal weight – forever! Ideally, you want to reach your ACE level when you're at your goal weight. So, adjust your carbs as needed to keep losing if you're not there yet. Many people end up with an ACE of between 65 and 100 grams of carbs. Some people might be considerably less and a few others could even higher.
- Maintain your control and your weight. Once you have found your ACE and before you move to phase 4 – Lifetime Maintenance – maintain your weight for a month. You can continue to introduce new foods once you don't go over your ACE. Again, pay close attention to how these new foods affect you if at all. This month is really the dress rehearsal for the Lifetime Maintenance phase.

How to do Phase 3 – Pre-Maintenance

- Add 10g of daily carbs every week or every few weeks. If you finished Phase 2 at with a CLL (Carbohydrate Level for Losing) of 45 grams of carbs, start Phase 3 with 55 grams of carbs a day. Then increase your daily carb intake every week or every few weeks by 10

- grams. If weight loss stalls or cravings return step back by 10g.
- Count carbs – you have probably gathered from the objectives above that you will need to write down what you eat and note the carb amounts. Otherwise you will really know how many grams of carbs you are eating and will not be able to discover your ACE. Again this will also let you identify easily if a new food is causing a problem.
- As you have done from the beginning, be sure that at least 12 to 15 grams of your total daily carb intake is made up of foundation vegetables – see the veg in Phase 1 of the Acceptable Food List for a list of over 50 of these along with tips on how to cook them and links to recipes.
- Add new foods one by one, following the Carb Ladder, starting with legumes, unless you've been able to reintroduce them in OWL—as vegetarians and vegans almost certainly have.
- Keep eating the recommended amounts of protein and sufficient natural fats to feel satisfied at the end of each meal.
- Continue to drink plenty of water and other acceptable beverages.
- Consume enough salt, broth, or soy sauce (unless you take diuretics) to avoid symptoms that may accompany the switch to fat-burning as long as your Net Carb intake is 50 grams or less. Two cups of Bovril a day will do the trick also. Once you exceed 50 grams of carbs this you won't need this.
- Take your multivitamin/multi mineral and omega-3 fatty acid supplements.
- Be sure to have your Atkins bars, shakes and treats on hand to prevent you from resorting to bad choices that might derail your progress.

What happens if I reach a plateau?

There's a good chance that at some point you reach a plateau and stop losing weight. The pace of weight loss is often erratic and many people lose weight in fits and starts. However, the definition of a plateau when you lose nothing despite doing everything for a period of at least four weeks. If you are losing centimeters but not weight, then this is not a true plateau and you should keep doing what you are doing. Hitting a plateau can be very frustrating but dealing patiently with it is crucial to your continued success. Try the following tips:

- Tighten up on recording everything you eat and the carb amounts – this can make a big difference.
- Count all your carbs including lemon juice, sweetners etc
- Decrease your daily intake of carbs by 10 grams. You may simply have stumbled on your ACE (i.e. the number of grams of carbs or maintaining your weight) early. Once weight loss resumes move up in 5 gram increments again.
- Find and eliminate hidden carbs in sauces, drinks and processed foods.
- Increase your activity level or try new activities – this works for some people but not all.
- Increase your fluid intake to at least 8 glasses of water a day.
- Cut back on artificial sweeteners, low-carb products and fruits other than berries.

Check your calorie intake. We do not usually count calories on Atkins but if you are doing everything to the letter and haven't lost weight in 4 weeks you may need to check your calories. You probably could guess that too many calories will slow down your weight loss, but here's a surprise—too few will slow down your metabolism and slow weight loss.

The numbers will vary depending on your height, age and metabolism but it should be within the following ranges:

- Women: 1,500–1,800 calories a day.
- Men: 1,800–2,000 calories per day.

If you've been consuming alcohol, cut back or abstain for now.

If none of these modifications makes the scales budge for a month, then you really are on a plateau. The only way to overcome it is to continue to eat right and wait. Your body and the scales will eventually comply.

Tips for Success

The top tip for success is to have patience and follow the process. Also remember why you want to lose weight and improve your health – write down your reasons if it helps. Doing this will get you to your goal weight and mean you know what you need in order to stay there. permanently!

Phase 4 – Maintenance

Congratulations! You have reached your ideal weight! It's a fantastic achievement – and a position that many many people who are overweight would like to be in. I'm sure clothes shopping or beach holidays are much more fun now! And hearing positive comments from people you haven't seen in a while!

You can be sure that your health markers are all telling a positive story too – if you had a check up before you started now would be a great time to do it again to see exactly how much those numbers have improved. You might well find that if you were on medication for high blood pressure, cholesterol or other conditions that these are no longer needed – check with your doctor. If you are diabetic, you should have been closely monitored by your doctor during this journey and have possibly already reduced if not eliminated your medications under their guidance. If you think back to before you started this journey, you have probably noticed many minor ailments or some not so minor have disappeared along this journey to the slim healthy new you.

Here are just some of the benefits that you need to know for the atkins diet phase 4:

- Improved cholesterol
- Lower triglycerides (these are a marker for heart disease)
- One diabetic reported blood sugar dropping from 7.9 to 3.9 – which is in the normal range
- Sleeping better
- Migraines gone
- Acne cleared up
- Painkillers not needed for PMS anymore
- Acid reflux gone – had been on 2 tablets a day for 15 years

- Bloated feeling after meals gone
- 'Mental fog' gone
- More energy
- No longer needs a nap in the afternoon
- Joint pain gone
- Improved self-esteem

Of course, these improvements often lead to improvements in other areas of life and business too. Many of these benefits kicked a mere week or two after starting Induction. However, human nature being what it is we tend to forget it after a while and feeling this good becomes the new normal, as it should. Now that you have reached Maintenance it is worth taking stock and thinking back on all the benefits you have gained with this way of life – both in terms of weight loss, health, vitality and general feel-good factor. This will help you with staying on this path and maintaining all of these benefits.

HOW TO DO PHASE 4 – MAINTENANCE

In Pre-Maintenance you learned what your ACE (Atkins Carbohydrate Equilibrium) was– this is the number of grams of carbs you can eat daily and neither gain or lose weight. All you need to do is continue to eat the way you've been eating in Pre-Maintenance, remaining at or just below your ACE.

For those with a high ACE:

If you have a high carbohydrate threshold and are physically active you are already eating foods from rungs 7 – 10 of the carbohydrate ladder. These would include starchy vegetables, fruit other than berries and whole grains – see the Atkins Carb ladder for more. As before when you introduce new foods, pay attention to how they make you feel and whether they weight gain, hunger or cause cravings to come back.

For those with an ACE below 50g:

If your carbohydrate threshold is below 50 grams of Net Carbs, you'll probably have to stay away from starchy vegetables, most fruit and whole grains or eat them rarely or in very small amounts. Exercising is one excellent way to increase you carbohydrate level and many people feel much more inclined to do so after they have lost some weight and have increased energy levels. Even if it turns out that your ACE is quite low – it's important to keep in mind that at least now you know what you need in order to maintain your weight and keep all those benefits we spoke about. After all the goal is to banish that extra weight forever – not win a competition for having the highest ACE possible!

You also know at this stage that there are lots of delicious meals you can enjoy no matter what your ACE. And as only someone who has followed this nutritional approach can understand, you know that giving up those refined carbs you used to eat for good is not at all a difficult prospect you imagined before beginning this way of eating. So it really is fantastic that you have learned what you need to stay slim and healthy forever – whatever the carb level.

What You Can Eat in Phase 4

In the Maintenance Phase your level of carbohydrates will essentially be the same as it was in Pre-Maintenance. Of course, you can re-introduce new foods in the months and years to come while staying below that carbohydrate level – as before be alert to see whether they cause weight gain or any other adverse effects.

Many people find that their appetite increases slightly as they approach their body's natural healthy weight even as they stay within their ACE. Now that you are no longer burning body fat for fuel it's important to understand that the extra fuel to keep your weight stable should come from dietary fat instead. In this way, your body stays in fat-burning mode. This is important so that you don't veer back to a state where your body burns carbs as it primary fuel – which brings back those blood sugar swings, poor energy and inevitably weight-gain. So if your weight drops below the desired level or you find that you are hungry you should also slightly increase good fats in your diet. To give you some ideas, you could add 3 – 5 portions of the following (as your appetite dictates) to your diet:

- 1 tablespoon of oil for dressing salads
- 1 tablespoon of butter
- 2 tablespoons of cream
- 5g cheese
- 10 large ripe olives with a teaspoon of olive oil
- Half an advocado
- 30g of almonds, walnuts, pecans or macadamias
- 1 tablespoon of full fat mayonnaise
- 2 tablespoons of pesto
- 2 tablespoons of nut butter

Hopefully by now, you are no longer afraid of fats (as many people are due the the fat-phobic advice we're all been given over the last 30 years) and you know that dietary fat is good for you in the context of a low carbohydrate diet. Your body at this stage is a very efficient fat-burning machine and these additions of fat in your diet will help keep your weight stable (as counter-intuitive as this might sound). The only dietary fat you should truly avoid are trans fats. An increased intake of trans fats is associated with an increased heart attack risk and inflammation in the body. They are typically found in foods you should be avoiding already, including fried foods, baked goods, biscuits, crackers, sweets, snack foods, icings and vegetable shortenings.

Phase 4 And The Rest of Your Life

Hopefully you understand by now that you will remain on phase 4 – the Lifetime Maintenance Phase – for the rest of your life! This makes sure the weight you have so successfully lost, stays lost forever! As we've said from the outset this diet is more of a lifestyle change and way-of-eating for life than a 'diet' you follow for a few weeks or months and then stop. If you go back to the way you used to eat, you will get the results you got the first time – weight gain and all that goes with it.

Of course we are not saying that you can't ever eat a slice of cake or the occasional slice of pizza. In the same way that some people are fine with alcohol in moderation, some people will find they can have these foods occasionally and it doesn't cause any problems. However, for others having just a little is the same as someone that can't handle alcohol – they find it much easier to avoid it completely and that it's just not worth the chance of eating these foods leading to a full-blown binge.

It is important to arrive at a place where you are mindful of your weight but not obsessed with it. Keep an eye on your weight and your measurements. Be alert to cravings coming back, unreasonable hunger or the return of any symptoms you had banished. Then take a look at what you have been eating. Maybe it was a case of carb creep or the effects or one or two recently added foods. Never let yourself gain more than 5 lbs without taking action to restore your goal weight. If this happens simply drop 10 to 20g of carbs and the weight should retreat. Or if need be, return to OWL for a week or two under it is under control again.

Keep in mind too that life events can affect your weight and cause you to slip:

You used to play a team sport but had an injury and had to stop

You had a baby and find yourself stressed and sleep deprived

Your doctor prescribes anti-depressants to help you deal with a family crisis

A new job means you need to travel more making it more difficult to keep up with you fitness regime and plan suitable meals

You suffer a disappointment or a break-up and this sends you back to your old unhealthy eating habits

You start a new relationship with someone who doesn't follow the Atkins diet

The key in all of these situations is to be mindful of these life changes and make adjustments to remain at your desired weight. There are lots of strategies you can take to deal with different life events so they don't derail the fantastic progress you've made and so that you achieve the ultimate goal of staying slim.

Chapter 4: Food List Of The Atkins Diet

If you're giving the Atkins diet a try, then you need to add these foods to your grocery list.

Atkins Diet List of Foods

If you're having trouble finding out what to make for dinner, there are plenty of Atkins diet recipes online and in print that include acceptable Atkins diet snacks and Atkins diet desserts. Don't have the time to find Atkins diet meal plans yourself? Just download the app for quick access to hundreds of daily meal options. Although there are several Atkins diet recipes on the actual Atkins site, here is a comprehensive list of all of the foods you can eat on the Atkins 20 Atkins diet plan.

Atkins Diet Phase 1

The Atkins diet Phase 1 (also known as the "induction" phase) list of acceptable foods includes:

- All fish, including: flounder, sole, herring, salmon, sardines, tuna, trout, cod, halibut.
- All fowl, including: Cornish hen, chicken, duck, goose, pheasant, quail, turkey, and ostrich.
- All shellfish, including: clams, crabmeat, mussels, oysters, shrimp, squid, and lobster. (Please note that oysters and mussels are higher in carbs, so if you're craving either, you should limit yourself to four ounces per day.)
- All meat, including: bacon, beef, ham, lamb, pork, veal, and venison. (Please note that some processed

meats, like bacon and ham, are cured with sugar. Check the package before indulging!)
- Any egg prepared in any style, including: deviled, fried, hard boiled, omelets, poached, scrambled, and soft-boiled.
- Fats (the good kind) and oils, including: butter, mayonnaise (with no added sugar), olive oil, vegetable oils, canola oil, walnut oil, soybean oil, sesame oil, grape seed oil, sunflower oil, safflower oil.
- Artificial sweeteners, including: sucralose, saccharin, and stevia.
- Beverages including: clear broth, bouillon (make sure there's no sugar added), club soda, cream (heavy or light), decaffeinated or regular coffee and tea, diet soda (take note of the carb count, which should be zero), flavored seltzer (no-calorie seltzer only), herb tea (without added barley or fruit sugar), unflavored soy/almond milk, and water (eight ounces per day). Water options include filtered water, mineral water, spring water, and tap water.
- Cheese, including: Parmesan (grated), goat, cheddar, gouda, mozzarella (whole milk), cream cheese (whipped), Swiss, and feta. (Cheese is an amazing thing, but it does contain carbs, so you should stick to three to four ounces of cheese per day.)
- Foundation vegetables, including: alfalfa sprouts, chicory greens, endives, escaroles, olives (green and black), watercress, arugula, radishes, spinach, bok choy, lettuce, turnip greens, hearts of palm, radicchio, artichoke, celery, collard greens, pickles, broccoli rabe, sauerkraut, avocados, daikon radish, red and white onions, zucchini, cucumbers, cauliflower, beet greens, broccoli, fennel, okra, rhubarb, swiss chard, asparagus, broccolini, bell peppers, sprouts, eggplants, kale, scallions, turnips,

tomatoes, jicama, portobello mushrooms, yellow squash, cabbage, green beans, leeks, shallots, brussel sprouts, cherry tomatoes, spaghetti squash, kohlrabi, pumpkin, snow peas, and garlic. (During Phase 1, you should be eating roughly 12 to 15 grams of net carbs per day in the form of vegetables. This high-fat, high-protein, and low-carb introduction will give you a solid kick start.)
- Salad garnishes, including: crumbled bacon, hard-boiled egg, sauteed mushrooms, sour cream, and grated cheeses.
- Herbs and spices, including: basil, cayenne pepper, cilantro, dill, oregano, tarragon, parsley, chives, ginger, rosemary, sage, black pepper, and garlic.
- Salad dressings, including: red wine vinegar, caesar, ranch, lemon juice, blue cheese, lime juice, balsamic vinegar, Italian, and creamy Italian.

Atkins Diet Phase 2

Below is the Atkins diet Phase 2 (also known as the "Balancing" phase) list of acceptable foods (this list, plus the items listed above). You'll be allowed to add higher carbs into your diet during Phase 2 (think nuts and fruits).

- Dairy, including: mozzarella cheese, yogurt (Greek and plain), unsweetened milk, whole milk, ricotta cheese, cottage cheese, and heavy cream.
- Nuts and seeds, including: Brazil nuts, macadamias, hulled sunflower seeds, walnuts, almonds, pistachios, peanuts, pecans, and cashews.
- Fruits, including: blackberries, raspberries, cranberries, strawberries, cantaloupe, honeydew, gooseberries, boysenberries, and blueberries.
- Juices, including: lemon juice, lime juice, and tomato juice.

- Beans, including: lentils, kidney beans, lima beans, pinto beans, black beans, navy beans, great northern beans, and chickpeas.

Atkins Diet Phase 3

Below is the Atkins diet Phase 3 (also referred to as the "Fine-Tuning" phase) list of acceptable foods (this list, plus the items listed above):

- Starchy vegetables, including: carrots, rutabaga, beets, acorn squash, sweet potatoes, parsnips, potatoes, and corn.
- Fruit, including: coconut, figs, cherries, watermelon, pomegranate, papayas, plums, guava, apples, clementines, grapefruit, kiwis, apricots, pineapple, peaches, mangoes, grapes, oranges, dates, bananas, and pears.
- Grains, including: wheat bran, wheat germ, oat bran, quinoa, whole-wheat bread, oatmeal, polenta, grits, whole-wheat pasta, barley, millet, and rice.

Once you've reached Phase 4, you've learned which foods boost the metabolism and which foods you should avoid. All of the "acceptable" foods in the fourth phase of the Atkins diet overlap with the foods listed in Phase 3, so you shouldn't have any problem transitioning.

Atkins Diet Phase 4

Below is the Atkins diet Phase 4 (also known as the "Maintenance" phase) list of acceptable foods (this list, plus the items listed above):

- Starchy vegetables including: carrots, rutabaga, beets, peas, acorn squash, butternut squash, sweet potatoes, parsnips, potatoes, and corn.
- Fruit, including: coconuts, figs, cherries, watermelon, pomegranate seeds, papayas, plums, raisins, guava, clementines, apples, kiwis, grapefruit, apricots, pineapples, peaches, mangoes, grapes, oranges, dates, bananas, and pears.

- Grains, including: wheat bran, wheat germ, oat bran, quinoa, whole-wheat bread, oatmeal, polenta, grits, whole-wheat pasta, barley, millet, and rice.

Chapter 5: Breakfast Recipes

ALMOND AND COCONUT MUFFIN

Ingredients

- 2 tablespoons Almond Meal Flour
- 1 teaspoon Coconut flour, high fiber
- 1 teaspoon Sucralose Based Sweetener (Sugar Substitute)
- 1/2 teaspoon Cinnamon
- 1/4 teaspoon Baking Powder (Straight Phosphate, Double Acting)
- 1/8 teaspoon Salt
- 1 large Egg
- 1 teaspoon Extra Virgin Olive Oil
- 1 tablespoon Sour Cream

Instructions

1) Place all dry ingredients in a coffee mug. Stir to combine.
2) Add the egg, oil, and sour cream. Stir until thoroughly combined.
3) Microwave for 1 minute. Use a knife if necessary to help remove the muffin from the cup, slice, butter, eat. For best results, eat immediately.

Note: Almond Meal from whole almonds is preferred for this recipe. Your MIM can be toasted once it's cooked and topped with cream cheese if you like. Replace the cinnamon with other spices, sugar-free syrup or 1/2 tsp unsweetened cocoa (net carb count will be .2g higher). Change the shape by making it in a bowl.

Almond-Pineapple Smoothie

INGREDIENTS

- 1/2 cup (8 fluid ounces) Plain Yogurt (Whole Milk)
- 2 1/2 ounces Pineapple
- 20 each wholes Blanched & Slivered Almonds
- 1/2 cup Pure Almond Milk - Unsweetened Original

INSTRUCTIONS

Feel free to substitute other fruits or nuts for the pineapple and/or almonds (about 20 whole almonds, 3 Tbsp slivered). Be sure to use fresh pineapple in this smoothie. Canned pineapple is swimming in sugar.

Combine the yogurt, pineapple, almonds and almond milk in a blender and purée until smooth and creamy.

Atkins Pancakes

INGREDIENTS

- 1 individual packet Sucralose Based Sweetener (Sugar Substitute)
- 2 teaspoons Baking Powder (Straight Phosphate, Double Acting)
- 1/4 teaspoon Salt
- 1 large Egg (Whole)
- 1 cup Cream (Half & Half)
- 3 servings Atkins Flour Mix

INSTRUCTIONS

Blend together 1 cup baking mix, sugar substitute, baking powder and salt in a large mixing bowl.

Add the half and half and egg. Whisk batter. Let the mixture sit for at least 5 minutes to activate the baking powder.

Coat the griddle with olive oil spray. Over medium heat, cook 4 pancakes at a time. When bubbles appear on the top and the edges are firm, flip the pancakes and cook another 2-3 minutes. Keep warm in the oven.

Repeat with remaining pancakes.

Baked Eggs and Asparagus

- 8 spear, small (5" long or less) Asparagus
- 1/4 cup Heavy Cream
- 2 large Eggs (Whole)
- 2 tablespoons Almond Meal Flour
- 1 tablespoon Parmesan Cheese (Shredded)
- 1/8 teaspoon Garlic
- 1/8 teaspoon Black Pepper

INSTRUCTIONS

Preheat oven to 400°F. Prepare a small oven safe casserole or 4-inch by 3-inch dish with a little bit of oil. Set aside.

Boil the asparagus spears for 2 minutes until tender-crisp. Drain and run under cold water then pat dry. Arrange in the prepared baking dish.

Pour cream over the asparagus and then crack two eggs on top.

In a small bowl blend together the almond meal, Parmesan cheese, garlic and black pepper. Sprinkle over the eggs and place in the oven. Cook for 5-10 minutes depending upon how you like your eggs cooked. Longer time will result in a firmer yolk. The cream will puff over the edges of the eggs and the topping should be golden brown and fragrant.

Atkins Waffles

INGREDIENTS

- 1 individual packet Sucralose Based Sweetener (Sugar Substitute)
- 1 large Egg (Whole)
- 2 teaspoons Baking Powder (Straight Phosphate, Double Acting)
- 1/4 teaspoon Salt
- 1 cup Cream (Half & Half)
- 3 servings Atkins Flour Mix

INSTRUCTIONS

Use the Atkins recipe to make Atkins Flour Mix for this recipe. This recipe makes 5 waffles. Assuming your waffle iron makes 4 servings, use four-fifths of the batter and then make a single waffle with the remaining batter. Freeze extra waffles and just pop in the toaster before serving.

In a large bowl, blend together 1 cup baking mix, baking powder, sugar substitute and salt.

In another large bowl, mix the half-and-half and beaten egg.

Add dry ingredients to the liquid ingredients and whisk batter until any lumps are removed. Don't overbeat.

Let the mixture sit for at least 5 minutes to activate the baking powder.

Heat the waffle iron and pour the batter in the center of the waffle iron.

Close the top and cook waffles for about 1 1/2 minutes or until golden brown.

Repeat with last waffle.

ATKINS DIET

Easier to Follow than Keto, Paleo, Mediterranean or Low-Calorie Diet, Allows You to Lose Weight Quickly, Without Saying Goodbye to Super Prohibited Sweets & Ice Cream in a Diet (Part 2)

BY

Jessica Davidson

© Copyright 2020 - All rights reserved.

The content contained within this book may not be reproduced, duplicated or transmitted without direct written permission from the author or the publisher.
Under no circumstances will any blame or legal responsibility be held against the publisher, or author, for any damages, reparation, or monetary loss due to the information contained within this book. Either directly or indirectly.

Legal Notice:
This book is copyright protected. This book is only for personal use. You cannot amend, distribute, sell, use, quote or paraphrase any part, or the content within this book, without the consent of the author or publisher.

Disclaimer Notice:
Please note the information contained within this document is for educational and entertainment purposes only. All effort has been executed to present accurate, up to date, and reliable, complete information. No warranties of any kind are declared or implied. Readers acknowledge that the author is not engaging in the rendering of legal,

financial, medical or professional advice. The content within this book has been derived from various sources. Please consult a licensed professional before attempting any techniques outlined in this book.

By reading this document, the reader agrees that under no circumstances is the author responsible for any losses, direct or indirect, which are incurred as a result of the use of information contained within this document, including, but not limited to, — errors, omissions, or inaccuracies.

Introduction

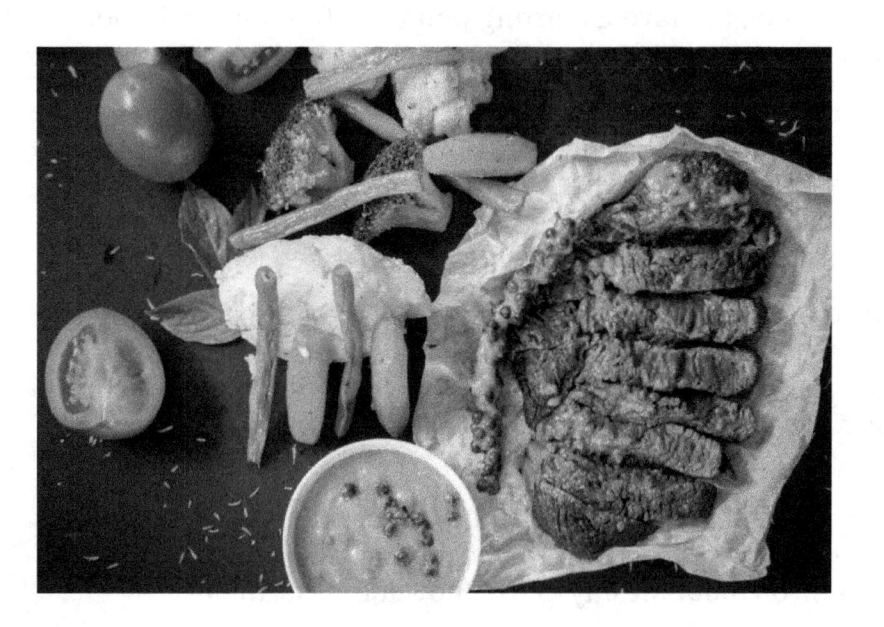

An Introduction to ATKINS Diet

What is Atkins Diet?

The Atkins Diet was created by Dr. Robert Atkins, a cardiologist whose interest in the health benefits of low-carb diets first culminated in the 1972 book "Dr. Atkins Diet Revolution," The diet involves four phases, starting with very few carbs and eating progressively more until you get to your desired weight.

In phase one, for example, you're allowed 20 grams a day of "net carbs," 12 to 15 of them from "foundation vegetables" high in fiber like arugula, cherry tomatoes and Brussels sprouts, according to the traditional Atkins 20 plan. This is advised for maximum weight loss. Two other iterations of the diet, Atkins 40, which the company says is "perfect for those who have less than 40 pounds to lose," and Atkins 100, a plan promoted to those seeking to maintaining their current weight, have a starting point of 40 grams and 100 grams of net carbs per day, respectively.

Generally speaking, the theory is that by limiting carbs, your body has to turn to an alternative fuel – stored fat. So sugars and "simple starches" like potatoes, white bread and rice are all but squeezed out; protein and fat like chicken, meat and eggs are embraced. Fat is burned; pounds come off.

But reducing total carbs isn't all there is to Atkins. Limiting the carbs you take in at any one time is also in the game plan. A carb-heavy meal floods the blood with glucose, too much for the cells to use or to store in the liver as glycogen. Where does it end up? As fat.

In terms of plan flexibility, Atkins 100 allows you to eat the widest variety of foods in the beginning, allocating 100 net carbs throughout the day. Here's how it breaks down:

- A minimum of 12 to 15 grams of net carbs a day of foundation vegetables
- Three 4- to 6-ounce servings of protein a day
- Two to four servings of added fat a day

The remaining 85 grams of net carbs come from foods like legumes, nuts or seeds, higher-carb fruits and vegetables and whole grains.

Low-Carb Diet

These diets provide fewer carbs than is recommended by government guidelines and are known to bring on quick weight loss.

How much does Atkins Diet cost?

Meat and fresh veggies are pricier than most processed and fast foods, so the Atkins Diet is typically more expensive than the average American's. How much more than usual you'll spend will depend largely on your choices of protein sources. Are you buying mostly ground beef or springing for veal? Chicken or turkey? Chuck vs. New York strip? Buying in season should keep the veggie tab reasonable.

Will Atkins Diet help you lose weight?

Atkins and other low-carb diets have been studied longer and harder than most other approaches, and Atkins does appear to be moderately successful, especially in the first couple of weeks. That's only part of the story, however.

Much of the initial loss is water, say experts, because of the diet's diuretic effect. That's true of many other diets, too, and is one of the reasons researchers don't judge diets based on a few weeks of results. In diet studies, long-term generally starts at two years. Here's what several key studies had to say about Atkins and other low-carb diets:

Over short periods, Atkins results vary. In one study, published in 2006 in the British Medical Journal, Atkins dieters lost an average of 10 pounds in the first four weeks while those on meal-replacement (Slim Fast), caloric-restriction (Weight Watchers) and low-fat (Rosemary Conley's "Eat Yourself Slim" book) diets lost 6 to 7 pounds. At the one-month point and thereafter, however, there were no significant differences in weight loss among the groups.

A 2007 study that appeared in the Journal of the American Medical Association divided roughly 300 overweight or obese women into groups and assigned them to one of four types of diets: low-carb (Atkins), low-fat (Ornish), low saturated-fat/moderate-carb (LEARN), and roughly equal parts protein, fat, and carb (Zone). At two months, the Atkins dieters had lost an average of about 9½ pounds compared with 5 to 6 pounds for those on the other three diets. At six months, weight loss for the Atkins group averaged about 13 pounds; the other three groups averaged 4 1/2 to 7 pounds. At 12 months, the Atkins group had lost what researchers called a "modest" 10 pounds; the other dieters averaged 3 1/2 to 6 pounds. Drawing firm conclusions from this study is risky, however. The dropout rate in all four groups was significant, and many participants didn't follow their assigned diet. The Atkins dieters, for example, took in far more carbs than they were supposed to.

A third study, published in 2010 in the Annals of Internal Medicine, found no clear advantage either to a low-carb diet based on Atkins or a generic low-fat diet. Both helped participants lose an average of 11% of their starting weight at 12 months, but they gained about a third of it back after that. At two years, average loss for both diets was 7% of initial body weight. (That's still not bad – if you're overweight, losing just 5 to 10% of your current weight can help stave off some diseases.) An analysis of five studies that compared low-carb and low-fat diets published in 2006 in the Archives of Internal Medicine concluded similarly – while weight loss was greater at six months for low-carb dieters, by 12 months that difference wasn't significant.

It is still unclear, regardless of claims made for low-carb diets, whether the main reason for weight loss is carb restriction specifically or simply cutting calories. A study published in 2009 in the New England Journal of Medicine found that after two years, participants assigned either to a 35% or a 65% carb diet lost about the same amount of weight – 6 to 7 1/2 pounds on average. In 2003, researchers who analyzed about 100 low-carb studies concluded in the Journal of the American Medical Association that weight loss on those diets was associated mostly with cutting calories and not with cutting carbs.

Researchers reviewed 17 different studies that followed a total of 1,141 obese patients on low-carb eating plans, some similar to the Atkins diet. Results were published in 2012 in Obesity. The study shows that low-carb dieters lost an average of nearly 18 pounds over a period of six months to a year. They also saw improvements in their waist circumference.

In a study published in November 2014 in Circulation: Cardiovascular Quality and Outcomes, researchers analyzed existing research on Atkins, South Beach, Weight Watchers and the Zone diets to find out which was most effective. Their findings suggested that none of the four diet plans led to significant weight loss, and none was starkly better than the others when it came to keeping weight off for a year or more. Each of the four plans helped dieters shed about the same number of pounds in the short term: around 5% of their starting body weight. After two years, however, some of the lost weight was regained by those on the Atkins or Weight Watchers plans. Since the diets produce similar results, the study authors concluded that dieters should choose the one that best adheres to their lifestyle – for example, Weight Watchers involved a group-based, behavior-modification approach, and Atkins focuses on lowering carbs.

Following the Atkins Diet will likely seriously challenge your willpower. How much do you love sweet and starchy foods? Would you miss crusty French bread? Pasta? Grape jelly? Diets that severely limit entire food groups for months and years tend to have lower success rates than less-restrictive diets do, and the Atkins Diet is the definition of a restrictive diet.

One study showed higher percentages of Atkins dieters dropping out at three, six, 12 and 24 months than others did on a low-fat diet, but the differences were not significant. Two other studies that included low-carb dieters concluded diet type wasn't connected to dropout rate.

The Atkins Diet isn't known for its convenience. At home, building variety into meals is a little harder than usual. Eating out takes more effort. Alcohol is limited. Company products and online resources may be helpful. In 2013, Atkins launched a frozen-food line, which the company says is the first low-carb frozen-food line on the market.

Atkins recipes abound. Atkins provides meal plans, recipes with ingredient lists and food carb counts, all in print-friendly format. There is at least a smattering of recipes across a range of cuisines from American to Middle Eastern to French to Asian.

Eating out is doable on the Atkins Diet. Just make sure you've read Atkins' list of approved fast-food and cuisine-specific options before heading out (and don't be bashful about asking lots of questions about meal preparation).

Chapter 6:
Hitting the Diet Bottom

I just can't get on with another diet plan; you are my last resort." Sandra has been on a diet her entire existence and has understood that she could no longer support a single diet program. She had been with all of them, Atkins, Dukan, The Area, South Beach, grapefruit diet ... too many diets for the details. Sandra was a professional on a diet. Initially, the diet was fun, even stimulating. "Usually, I thought this diet will be different right now." So the routine would be reloaded with every fresh diet, every summer. But the lost weight would eventually be recovered as an undesirable tax bill.

Sandra had hit bottom in the diet plan. At this point, however, I was even more obsessed with meals and her body than ever. She felt silly. "I would have managed and controlled this in the past." What he did not understand was that the dietary procedure had been carried out. Dieting made her even more worried about meals. Diet had made enemy meals. The acquired diet made his experience guilty when he did not consume dietary foods (although she was not officially on a diet). Dieting experienced slowed her metabolism.

Sandra took years to understand that the diet does not work (yes, she knew the emerging idea that the diet does not work, but usually thought it would be different). Some experts and consumers recognize the premise that fast diets don't work: it is difficult for a country of people who are enthusiastic about their bodies to think that even a "practical diet" is often useless. Sandra has been hooked by the interpersonal mythology of the modern age group, the "great hope of diet", for most of her lifestyle since her first diet program at the age of fourteen.

At thirty, Sandra felt trapped: she still wanted to lose weight and was uncomfortable in her body. While Sandra couldn't bear the very thought of another diet plan, she didn't understand that the majority of her food problems were actually due to her dieting. Sandra was also discouraged and angry-"I understand everything about diets." Certainly, she could recite calorie consumption and fat grams, just like a walking dietary data source. This is the big warning of losing excess weight and avoiding it usually isn't a problem of understanding. If all we had to have a normal weight was to understand food and nutrition, most people in the United States would not be overweight. The information is easily available. (Take any women's magazine, and you will find abundant diet plans and comparisons with meals).

In addition, the more you try to follow the diet, the more you will fall (it certainly hurts to never succeed in case you have done the best). The best description due to this effect is distributed by John Foreyt, Ph.D., one of the leading professionals of diet psychology. He compared it to a Chinese puzzle (the hollow straw cylindrical puzzle, in which an index finger is placed on each end). The more you try to get out, the more pressure you will exert, the harder it will be to escape the puzzle. Instead, you find yourself locked up in a narrower place ... caught ... frustrated.

Symptoms of Diet Plan Backlash
Diet backlash may be the cumulative side-effect of dieting-it could be short-term or chronic, depending on how long one has been dieting. It can only be one or more side effects. When Sandra got to any office, she already had the traditional symptoms of a violent reaction to the diet. Not only was she tired of following a diet, but she ate less food, but she also had problems losing weight during her new diet

attempts. Additional symptoms include:

a. The simple contemplation of starting a diet causes desires and cravings for "sinful" and "fatty" foods, such as ice cream, chocolate, biscuits, etc.
b. When you quit a diet, go overeating and feel guilty. One research indicated that post- dieting binges happen in 49 per cent of most individuals who end a diet.
c. Have low self-esteem with meals. It's understandable that every diet program taught you never to trust the body or the food you dedicate. Although it may be the procedure for the diet that fails, failure continues to undermine its romantic relationship with food.
d. Since you don't deserve to consume because you're overweight.
e. Reduced duration of the diet. Living on a diet is getting shorter. (It could be indisputable that the Ultra Slim-Fast sales page is "Give us weekly ... and we ..."
f. Last dinner. All diet plans are preceded by foods that you presume not to eat anymore. Food consumption often increases during this period. It can happen with a meal or in a few days. The last supper seems to be the last step before the "nutritional cleansing", almost a farewell party. For a single customer, Marilyn, each meal seemed to be the last. I ate every meal until it filled up uncomfortable since I was terrified that I would never eat again. Once for all reasons! He was on a diet because the first grade exceeded two-thirds of his existence! He experienced provisional fasting intervals and a series of low-calorie diets. As for his body, the diets were just around the corner, so it's best to eat when you can. Any food for Marilyn was a relief from hunger.
g. Social abstinence. Since it is difficult to go on a diet and visit a party or go out for dinner, it is easier to

refuse social invitations. At first, social avoidance of food may seem wiser for dieting reasons, but it becomes a big deal. There is often the concern of being able to maintain static control. It is not unusual for this meeting to be strengthened by "maintaining calorie intake or excess grams of fat for the party", which often means eating almost nothing. But by enough time the dieter finds the party, ravenous food cravings dominates and consuming feels very uncontrollable.

h. Sluggish metabolism. Each diet plan shows your body to adjust better to another purposeful starvation (another eating routine arrangement). The digestion backs off as the body utilizes each calorie successfully, as though it were the last. The more extreme the eating routine, the more it will push your body into the endurance condition that diminishes calories. Bolstering your digestion is like filling a fire. Expel the strong wood, and the fire diminishes. Essentially, to build the pace of digestion, we should eat a satisfactory measure of calories; generally, our life structures will redress and back off.

i. Use caffeine to endure the day. Espresso and diet drinks will, in general, be manhandled as a supervisory group to feel fiery while eating pretty much nothing.

j. Eating disorder. At long last, for a few, the rehashed diet is generally the foundation of a dietary problem (going from anorexia nervosa or bulimia to impulsive indulging).

Despite the fact that Sandra felt she could never again follow dieting, she was as yet engaged with the most recent wonder of the Supper. (We frequently meet him each time we see somebody just because.) Truth be told, she ate higher nourishment levels than expected and ate huge numbers of her preferred nourishments (he figured he could never observe these kinds of nourishment again). It seems as though you are arranging a long outing and planning additional garments. The straightforward thought of concentrating on her eating issues put her in the attitude of the pre-diet plan, something normal.

While Sandra essentially started to comprehend the worthlessness of the dieting, she should be slim had not changed, obviously a predicament. She clung to the appeal of honourable American want.

The Paradox of Dieting
Inside our general public, the quest for slenderness (both for wellbeing and physical make-up) has wound up being the call to war of clearly all Americans. Eating an individual nibble of any nourishment that is high in fat or non-healthfully redeemable is generally deserving of a "blameworthy" expression by affiliation. You may be paroled, in any case, for "extraordinary conduct." Good conduct, inside our way of life, implies beginning a crisp eating routine or having incredible aims to abstain from food. Along these lines starts the hardship routine of dieting - the battle of the "bulge and indulge". Rice cakes for seven days, Häagen-Dazs the following.

"I feel remorseful essentially for enabling the staple worker to perceive what I purchase," said another client, who by chance had his trolley loaded with a natural product, vegetables, entire grains, pasta and a little 16 ounces of genuine dessert. It seems as though we were in a state of utilization of the Food Law coordinated by the nourishment mafia. Furthermore, there consistently is by all accounts dieting you can't refuse. Embellishment? No. We are sensible for this discernment.

A report distributed in 1993 in Eating Disorders-The Journal of Treatment and Avoidance found that somewhere in the range of 1973 and 1991, notices for dietary guides (diet nourishments, nourishment decrease helps, and diet programs) expanded practically direct. The analysts likewise referenced that there is absolutely a parallel model at the beginning of utilization issue. It is speculated that the weight of the push on the dietary arrangement (through publicizing spots) for the most part importantly affects the pattern of buyer unsettling influence.

The dieting pressure plan is powered past TV ads. Magazine articles and film content add to the weight of being thin. Fragile cigarette announcements additionally go for the heaviness of the Achilles female heel with titles like Ultra Thin 100, Virginia Slims, and so forth. A Kent cigarette, "Thin Lights", explicitly portrays this push on ladies' physical issues. Your promotion is like that of an industrialist for a decrease in normal weight contrasted with a cigarette, featuring lean depictions: "long", "slight", "light". Obviously, the examples in cigarette ads are especially unpretentious. Obviously, the inside for disease control (CDC) traits and expansion in ladies' smoking to their need to be more slender. Tragically, we have heard ladies ponder in our workplaces who have likewise viewed as smoking again as a guide to getting more fit.

Be that as it may, weight reduction isn't only a worry of ladies (albeit clearly there is extra weight on ladies). The multiplication of business contributions of light lager has planted the seed of body mindfulness in men's considerations; in addition, a fit stomach is desirable over one of brew. It is no occurrence that we have seen the dispatch of magazines focused on men, for example, Males Fitness and Female's Health.

While the quest for slenderness has crossed the sexual orientation boundary, we have sadly brought forth the original of weight onlookers — an upsetting pattern towards new dieting influences the wellness of American youngsters.

Stunning exploration has shown that school-age kids are fixating on their weight-an impression of a nation eager about dieting and overabundance weight. The nation over, six-year-olds are getting thinner, scared of putting on weight, and being continuously treated for utilization issue that compromises their wellbeing and development protection. Social strain to shed pounds has bombed in kids. Not exclusively can eating less junk food work; it is generally the principle issue. Albeit many may follow dieting as a push to lose abundance weight or for wellbeing reasons, the conundrum is clearly that it could cause more damage. This is the thing that our nation must show to the eating routine:

a. Obesity is greater than any time in recent memory in grown-ups and youngsters.
b. Dietary problems are on the ascent.
c. Child weight issues have multiplied in the previous ten years.
d. Despite the way that there are still more without fat and dietary nourishments than previously, just about 66% of grown-ups are hefty or fat.
e. More than one thousand 200 and a lot of fat has just been liposuction from 1982 to 1992. (And as of late accessible review indicated that once a year after a liposuction procedure, fat returned, yet in another area of the body).
f. Diet builds the possibility to increase significantly a greater number of pounds than you have lost!

Dieting Intake Cannot Battle Biology
Diet is a kind of transient yearning. Accordingly, when you are given a principal chance to eat truly, you experience so firmly that you feel wild, an edgy demonstration. With respect to natural yearning, all expectations to design the eating routine and the need to get in shape are temporary and incomprehensibly superfluous. In those concise

minutes, we become simply like the voracious man-expending plant in the film Little Store of Horrors, testing to eat-"Feed me, feed me."

While outrageous eating may appear to be crazy and unnatural, it is really a standard reaction to yearning and diet. Notwithstanding, it can frequently be viewed as that eating after the dieting doesn't have "determination" or imperfection in character. Be that as it may, in translating the post-dietary nourishment plan accordingly, it gradually disintegrates fearlessness with nourishment, diet after eating routine. Each infringement of the eating routine arrangement, each nourishment situation that appears to be wild establishes the frameworks for the "diet plan mindset", step by step and diet by diet. The evidently daring arrangement invest more energy following time-transforms into as dumbfounding as the Chinese finger confound. You can't fight science. At the point when your body starves, it should be bolstered. In any case, frequently a weight watcher gripes: "Just on the off chance that I experience determination." Clearly, this isn't just a self-control issue. (In spite of the fact that the splendid tribute from fat misfortune treatment focuses support this lost blame in determination.) When you are not encouraged, you will get fixated on nourishment, regardless of whether on a purposeful eating routine or craving.

You can't count calories, yet eat cautiously for the sake of wellbeing. This is by all accounts the politically right term for "diet" during the 90s. Be that as it may, in any event, for some, it's a similar issue with dinners, with similar side effects. Keeping away from overabundance fats or sugars, whatever occurs, and subsisting on basically sans fat or starch-free nourishments is basically an eating routine and frequently brings about a lacking eating routine. There are numerous kinds of diets and different sorts of diets. We will investigate your dietary character and meet the Intuitive

Eater in the following part.

Diet Increases your Risk of Getting More Weight! On the off chance that dietary applications were to withstand a similar control as medications, open utilization probably won't be permitted. Envision, for instance, taking asthma to medicate, which improves relaxing for half a month; however, over the long haul; it exacerbates the lungs and relaxing. Will I truly follow an eating routine (a great supposed "reasonable eating routine"), in the event that I realized I could make you put on weight?

Here is a couple of calming research demonstrating that eating less junk food advances weight gain:

a. A gathering of UCLA specialists inspected thirty-one long haul investigated on eating less junk food and figured slimming down is a consistent indicator of overabundance weight gain-up to 66% of the individuals recovered more abundance weight than they dropped (Mann et al., 2007).
b. Research on almost seventeen thousand kids between the ages of nine and fourteen finished up: "... in the long haul, the weight-controlling eating routine isn't just ineffectual, yet could advance weight gain" (Field et al. 2003).
c. People on a high school diet had twice the same number of odds of being overweight than adolescents on dieting regarding a multiyear review. Specifically, toward the start of the examination, individuals on an eating routine don't gauge significantly more than their companions who don't follow dieting. This is a significant detail, provided that individuals on dieting weigh much more, it could be a component of perplexity (which would suggest extra factors, as opposed to counting calories, for example, genetics).

Epic research on more than 2,000 units of twins from Finland, matured 16 to 25 years matured indicated that consuming fewer calories itself, free of hereditary qualities, is impressively connected with quickened fat addition and expanded danger of getting stout (Pietilaineet et al. 2011). Dietary twins, who experienced a solitary purposeful health improvement plan, were just about a few times bound to be overweight than their non-dietary twin partner. Likewise, the plausibility of unreasonable overweight improved in a portion subordinate way with every dietary occasion.

Studies aside: what did your dietary experiences show you? Numerous people and individuals in the lab state their first dieting plan was straightforward: the pounds basically liquefied away. Yet, that first dietary experience could be the temptation trap, which starts the vain quest for weight decrease through eating routine. We state pointless on the grounds that our bodies are amazingly wise and designed for endurance.

Organically, your body experiences the dieting process predominantly in light of the fact that it is a sort of starvation. Your cells don't comprehend you are intentionally limiting your dinner admission. The body shifts into base endurance mode-digestion diminish, and nourishment needing heighten. What's more, with each diet plan, your body learns and adjusts, which prompts weight gain in expansion. Therefore, many people feel simply like they absolutely are a disappointment; however, it truly is eating less junk food which has bombed them.

Chapter 7: What Type of Eater Are You?

You can continue on a diet and not know! There are many types of eating styles that are actually unconscious types of dieting. Quite a few people have said these were not really on a diet plan- but upon nearer inspection of what and how they consume, they were dieting still!

A good example here's. Ted arrived because he wished to lose excess weight. He said that in his fifty years of life, he had previously only been on four serious diet programs. In examining the titles of publications at work (compulsory overeating texts, consumption of books on ailments, etc.), he said: "You use many serious complications in the diet ... well, I'm not just one of those. Obviously, Ted did not consider himself a dietician, who ate simply with care, but showed that it was an unconscious diet.

Although Ted had not followed an active diet, he was eating at a level where he had almost passed out in the afternoon. The reason: he had been unhappy with his weight! In the morning I chose an intense bicycle trip down a hill, for only an hour. I would go back and have breakfast for a bit. Lunch was usually a salad with iced tea (although it seems healthy, it is too low in carbohydrates). At dinner time, your body will scream for meals. Ted not only had a severe calorie deficit, but he also lacked carbohydrates. Nights become a food party! Ted had the idea that it was previously a "food volume" problem with a solid sweet tooth. The truth is that previously he had an unconscious mentality in the diet that biologically triggered his night diet and his pleasant tooth.

Even Alicia hadn't been on a conscious diet. She never came to lose pounds, but because she wanted to increase her vitality. During the initial program, it became clear that he had problems with food. So they asked him if he had done many diets. She seemed amazed. "How did you know I did billions of diets?" While Alicia claimed to be comfortable with her current fat, she was still at war with food; she did not trust herself with meals. It turns out that Alicia has been on a diet since she was a child. Although he hadn't officially followed a diet, he maintained (and expanded) a couple of dietary guidelines with each diet plan that almost paralyzed her ability to eat normally. We observe this at all times, the hangover from dieting: avoiding certain foods no matter what, feeling uncontrollable as soon as a "sinful" meals are eaten, sense guilty when self-imposed food guidelines are broken (such as for example "Thou shalt not really eat previous to 6 P.M."), and so forth.

The unconscious diet usually occurs in the type of meticulous eating habits. There can be an excellent line between feeding on for health insurance and dieting. Notice how actually the frozen diet plan foods such as for example, Lean Cuisine and Excess weight Watchers are placing their focus on health instead of a diet. As long as you participate in some form of the diet, the recipient will eliminate food and body concerns. Whether you are a conscious or unconscious person, the results of the medial side are similar, the diet again, the effect of the eyelashes. It seems like a period in which one eats cautiously, "blowing" it and spending penance with an increase in diet or extremely cautious consumption. In this chapter, we will explore the many diet/nutrition styles to help see what your position is now. Later, you will meet the Intuitive Eater and the intuitive style of food, and the perfect solution is to live without diet programs.

The Eating Personalities

To help you clarify your food design style (or diet), we have identified the following key types of eaters that feature distinctive food patterns: the careful eater, the one that makes a professional diet and the eater unconscious. These consuming personalities are exhibited even if they are not officially on a diet. It is possible to have significantly more than one consuming personality, although we find that there is commonly a dominant trait. The chances of your life can also influence or change your personality to eat. For example, a client, a tax attorney, was usually a careful eater, but during the fiscal period of the year, it became the chaotic unconscious eater.

It is possible that it occasionally possesses the intake characteristics described below in the three nuclei that feed on personality. Note this, and if your feed exists in one of these domains most of the time, it's a problem.

Review each character you eat and see which one best reflects your style. By understanding what your position is now, it will be easier to find out how to become an intuitive eater. For example, you may find that you have already been involved in a type of diet and have not even recognized it. Or you can discover features that, without knowing it, work against you.

The careful eater
Cautious consumers are those who tend to be attentive to the food they put into their bodies. Ted was a good example of a careful eater (per day). At the top, accurate eaters look like "ideal" eaters. They are highly aware of nutrition. Externally, they seem oriented towards health and fitness (noble characteristics admired and strengthened in our society).

Style
There is a selection of eating behaviours exhibited by Careful Eater. In an intense moment, Cautious Eater can be

distressed for every bite of food allowed in the body. Shopping trips are spent looking at meal labels. Eating out can indicate interrogating the waiter what's in the meals, how maybe the meals prepared-and obtaining assurances that the meals are prepared particularly to the Cautious Eater's liking (not often one speck of essential oil or other excess fat used). What's incorrect with this? Aren't label reading and assertive cafe ordering in the medical interests of some individuals? Of program! However, the difference could be the vigilante force and the ability to forget any defect related to the choice of consumption. Attentive eaters tend to consume less than normal and control the amount of food consumed.

The attentive eater can spend most of his waking hours planning another meal or snack, often worried about eating. Since Careful Eater is not officially on a diet, your brain punishes all the "harmful", fatty or sugary foods you eat. The Careful Eater can travel the fine line between sincerely thinking about health and eating carefully with respect to body image.

Sometimes, Careful Eater is driven by periods or events. For example, some careful eaters are meticulous during weekdays, to make sure they get their "ideal of consumption" to "show off" on the weekends or for the next party. But on weekends they happen 104 times a year: waste can be counterproductive with unwanted weight gain. Consequently, it is not uncommon for a cautious eater to think about starting a diet.

The Problem

There's nothing incorrect with being thinking about the well-being of the body. However, the problem occurs when diligent consumption (almost in contact with the militant) affects a healthy relationship with food and negatively affects the body. Prudent eaters, on closer inspection, resemble a delicate diet style. They can't be on a diet;

however, they look into every food scenario.

The Professional Dieter
People on a professional diet are easier to identify; they are on a perpetual diet. In general, they tried the latest commercial diet, the diet book or the trick to lose weight. Sometimes, the diet is performed in the form of fasting or "reduction". Professional Dieters understand a whole lot about portions of foods, calories, and "dieting methods," yet the cause they are usually on another diet plan is that the initial one never worked. Today, Professional Dieter can be amply trained in counting carbohydrate grams.

Style

People on a professional diet also have accurate food traits. The difference, however, is that people on a diet chronically, guiding the choice of meals to lose weight, not necessarily for health. When the dieter is not officially on a diet, he generally thinks about the next diet that can be started. He often wakes up wishing this is a good day, the fresh start.

While people on a professional diet have a lot of knowledge of diets, they don't serve them well. It is not uncommon to allow them to eat compulsively or participate in the consumption of the Last Supper as soon as a prohibited meal is eaten. This is because people on a chronic diet really believe that they will no longer eat this food; tomorrow I'm on a diet, tomorrow they start again with a clean slate. Better eat right now; it's the last opportunity. And in addition, the Professional Dieter gets discouraged at the futility of the vicious routine. Diet, lose weight, put on weight, intermittent binges, and back again to dieting.

The Problem

It's very difficult to live in this manner. The Yo-Yo diet helps make losing excess weight more difficult as well as eating healthy. Chronic lack of food usually causes overeating or periodic feeding. For some diet professionals, the frustration of losing weight intensifies so much that they can try laxatives, diuretics and weight loss supplements. And trigger that these "dietary aids" generally don't work, they could try extreme methods like chronic restriction, in the type of anorexia nervosa or bleeding (like nausea after a binge), in the type of bulimia. While anorexia and bulimia are multifactorial and have their roots in psychological problems, a growing body of research suggests that chronic diet is usually a common step towards an eating disorder. One study specifically found that when enough dieters reach the age of fifteen, they are eight times more likely to have problems with an eating disorder than people who don't go on a diet.

The Unconscious Eater
The Unconscious Eater is often engaged in a paired diet, which consists of eating and simultaneously doing another activity, such as watching television and eating, or eating and reading. Due to the subtleties and insufficient awareness, it can become problematic for a person to recognize this eating character. There are numerous subtypes of unconscious eaters.

The Chaotic Unconscious Eater
Live a life that is too often programmed, too busy, too many things you can do. The chaotic, consuming design is haphazard; whatever's obtainable will end up being grabbed -vending machine fare, junk food, it'll all perform. Food and diet tend to be vital to this person-just not really in the critical instant of the chaos. Chaotic eaters tend to be so busy putting out fires that have difficulty identifying biological cravings for food until it is fiercely voracious. And in addition, the chaotic eater will go extended periods of time without eating.

The Refuse-Not Unconscious Eater

They are vulnerable to the simple existence of food, regardless of whether they are hungry or full. The jars of sweets, the meals at the meetings, the food sitting on the kitchen counter, probably none of them will be overcome. However, most of the time, it is fair; consumers who do not refuse to consume are not aware of what they are consuming or how much they consume. For example, the Reject-Not Eater can actually pick up some candy on the way to the bathroom without being aware of it. Social outings that revolve around meals such as cocktails and festive buffets are particularly difficult for Refuse-Not Eater.

The Waste-Not Unconscious Eater
Evaluate meals in dollars. His / her eating travel is frequently influenced by getting just as much as they are able to your money can buy. Waste-Not Eater is particularly inclined to completely clean the plate (and also that of others). It is not unusual for a waste eater not to actually consume the leftovers of children or spouse.

The Unconscious Emotional Eater
They use food to manage emotions, especially unpleasant feelings such as stress, anger and loneliness. While Emotional Eaters look at their consuming as the problem, it's often a sign of a deeper concern. Consuming behaviours of the Emotional Eater can range between grabbing a bag of chips on stressful occasions to chronic compulsive binges of huge quantities of food.

The problem

Unconscious power, in its many forms, usually be a problem if it translates into persistent excessive consumption (which can simply occur if you are eating instead of being very alert).

Remember that somewhere between the first and last bite of meals is where the awareness period actually occurs. Like in

"Oh, it's all over!"

For example, have you ever bought a large package of candy in the movies and started consuming it, and then you find that your fingertips suddenly scratch themselves under the empty container? This is a simple type of unconscious feeding. But unconscious nutrition can also exist at an extreme level, in a relatively altered feeding condition. In this case, the individual is not attentive to what is consumed, why he has started eating, or how he knows about the taste of the food. That is zoning out with meals.

When your Eating Personality Works Against You
Finally, the food varieties of Careful Eater, Professional Dieter and Unconscious Eater become an inefficient feeding method, even if at the top they seem to be fine. The perfect solution is for the discouraged consumer: try more with a fresh diet! At first, the new diet seems stimulating and hopeful, but in the end, the family pounds return. The diet becomes more demanding, and even if you resume your basal consumption personality, you may feel more unpleasant than before. It is because internal dietary guidelines are strengthened with each diet plan. These meal rules often perpetuate the guilt emotions of consumption, even when you are not officially on a diet. Furthermore, the biological ramifications of the diet make it increasingly difficult to have a normal romantic relationship with meals. The Intuitive Eater character, however, can be an exception. It's the only feeding design that doesn't work against you and will help you end chronic diets and yo-yo weight fluctuations.

Intuitive Eater Introduction
Intuitive eaters march with their signs of internal hunger and eat regardless of what they choose without feeling guilty or an ethical dilemma. The intuitive eater can be an independent eater. However, it is increasingly difficult to

become an unaltered eater in today's health-conscious society considering the bombardment of communications on food, food and weight by advertisers, the press and medical researchers. When we explained the basic feeding characteristics of Intuitive Eater to its customers, it is surprising how often we will hear the answer: "This is how my partner eats." This or how my boyfriend eats. "When we ask what the person's weight and romantic relationship is with food, the answer is: "No problem!" Consider small children. Intuitive, natural eaters will be practically free of social messages about meals and body image. Toddlers possess innate wisdom of meals, in the event that you don't hinder it. They don't eat predicated on dieting guidelines or health, yet study after research shows that if you allow a toddler consumes spontaneously; he'll eat what he requirements when given free usage of food. (This is most likely the toughest point for a concerned mother or father to do- to release and trust that children have an innate capability to eat!)

This is true even when food for food, food for little tykes is apparently a father's nightmare. Experts found that calorie intake was highly variable in confirmed foods; However, it has been balanced over time. However, many parents assume that their children cannot properly regulate their diet. As a result, parents often adopt coercive strategies in an attempt to ensure that the child eats a nutritionally sufficient diet. But a previous study by Birch and his colleagues indicates that these control strategies are countered. In addition, Birch notes that "parents' attempts to regulate their children's feeding have been reported more regularly by obese adults than by normal-weight adults." Likewise, Duke University psychologist Philip Costanzo, PhD found that unwanted weight in school-age children was closely related to the level at which parents sought to limit their children's food. Actually, well-meaning parents hinder Intuitive Eating. Whenever a mother or father attempts to overrule a child's organic eating cues, the nagging problem gets worse, not better.

A parent, who feeds a kid every time a hunger signal is heard and who stops feeding when the infant demonstrates he's had enough, may play a robust role in the original development of Intuitive Feeding on. Indeed, the innovative role of the therapist and dietician offered by Ellyn Satter has shown that, in the event that the parents of obese children cool down and allow them to consume without the pressure of their parents, the children will ultimately eat much less. Why? The child begins to listen and understand his internal signs of hunger and satiety. The child also knows that he will use food.

According to Satter, "children deprived of food so that they can lose weight, worry about food, fear they don't have enough to eat and are susceptible to overeating if they get the chance." We have found that this is accurate for dieters too. Limited to adults, the intuitive drinking process has been buried over a long period, often years and years. Instead of relaxing a father's pressure, this decrease in pressure should be the result of inside and against the myth of society about dieting and distorted body worship.

Fortunately, we all have the natural ability to eat intuitively; It has simply been suppressed, especially with the diet. This book specializes in showing you exactly how to wake the intuitive eater in you.

How Your Intuitive Eater Gets Buried
As toddlers get yourself a little older, the mixed messages start to creep in-from the early influences of the Saturday morning food commercial, to the well-meaning mother or father who coaxes his kid to "Clean your plate." The assault won't stop if you're a kid. There are many external forces that impact our eating, that may include additionally bury Intuitive Eating.

Dieting
You have already seen the damage from a chronic diet, which includes, among others:

a. Increase in excessive consumption
b. Decreased metabolic rate.
c. Greater concern about meals.
d. Increase the emotions of deprivation.
e. A greater sense of failure
f. Reduced feeling of willpower.

This only serves to erode your confidence in food and prompts you to rely on external sources to guide your diet (one diet, one diet and enough time of the day, food rules, etc.). The more you head to external resources to "judge" if your consuming is in balance, the additional removed you feel from Intuitive Eating. Intuitive Eating depends on your inner cues and signals.

Eat Healthy Messages Or Die
Messages about healthy eating are everywhere, from nonprofit healthcare organizations to food companies promoting the medical benefits of their unique item. The inherent message? Everything you consume can improve your wellbeing. Conversely, take one incorrect move (bite), and you're one step nearer to the grave. Is usually this an exaggeration? No. For example, a 1994 press release published by the Harvard College of Public Health mentioned that the consumption of trans-fatty acids (inside margarine) could cause thirty thousand deaths each year in the United States due to cardiovascular disease. That sort of message can easily keep you feeling guilty for consuming the "incorrect" kind of meals and feeling puzzled in what you should eat.

Magazines and newspapers have also significantly increased their protection of food and well-being. A food publisher, Joe Crea, of an important metropolitan newspaper, the Orange County Register (California), said that in a period of six to 12 months (1987-1993) his stories about food multiplied by five. Of nearly eight hundred food stories, two hundred had been linked to health problems. Although there is absolutely no doubt that everything you eat can affect your health, exponential coverage of the press has been offered as a channel for the development of food paranoia in the purchaser, particularly in the diet. Joe Crea agrees: "Open the newspaper, visit a good story about cheesecake and, at the same time, another piece on how eating too much will make you gain weight. Place the incompatible player.

Are we saying you should ignore the virtues of healthy intake? Of course not. However, if you have a diet adapted to your diet, the burst of "healthy eating" messages can make you feel more guilty about the foods you choose to eat. Obesity and Wellness reported a study of 2,075 adults in Florida that revealed that 45% of adults felt guilty after eating the foods they liked. (Remember that this study was carried out to reflect common American demographics. These "guilt-by- eating" figures would probably be higher if performed on dieters.)

Women could be particularly guilty. A Gallup poll by the American Dietetic Association showed that women feel more guilty than men for the foods they eat (44 per cent versus 28 per cent). Could this be because females diet more often than men? Or because ladies are usually the prospective of health communications and food advertisements (consider the number of women's magazines). Women will be primarily responsible for decisions relating to family health care and will often also be responsible for food and nutritional problems; They serve as the main objective.

We have found that establishing a healthy diet or diet as a short priority in the intuitive feeding process is counterproductive. We initially ignore nutrition, as it interferes with the relearn process of an intuitive eater. Nutrition heresy? No. Food can be respected and honoured. It simply cannot be the first priority when you've been on a diet for a lifetime. Or consider it this way; in case you have focused all your attention on the diet, does it help you? The many nutritious diet programs (absolute) may become embraced as another type of diet.

Chapter 8: Intuitive Eating Standards: Summary

Just once he vows to dispose of the diet and supplant it with an activity focused on intuitive nourishing, is he considering escaping jail from abundance weight variances and food fixations? In this part, we will present the fundamental ideas of intuitive sustaining: a preview of every idea, with an examination study or two. The most significant aftereffect of every customer referenced was that of acquiring a sound association with dinners and their bodies. By following ten intuitive eating ideas, you will standardize your sentimental association with food. A focus on weight reduction must be set aside for later. On the off chance that your present pounds offer came about because of getting withdrawn together with your inward insight about eating, and subsequently, of tuning back into this intelligence, weight reduction happens, along these lines be it. Assuming, by the by, you are as of now keeping your set point fat through the action of limiting, overeating, confining, and so forth, at that point, it truly is particularly essential that you put weight to decrease on the storage compartment burner.

Guideline One:

Declines the Mentality of the Dietary Plan
Dispense with diet books and magazine articles that give you the bogus any desire for getting more fit rapidly, effectively and for all time. Feel furious about the falsehoods that made you sense that you had flopped each time a new

diet quit working and you recovered all your weight. On the off chance that you enable a little want to demand that a crisp and better diet might be hiding close by, it will keep you from abstaining from rediscovering the intuitive diet.

For quite a while, we have sought after one diet plan for another, enabling the most stylish trend to direct what, how much, and when to eat. This inflexible way of life of limitation and hardship can bring about a dangerous association with food. The initial step on the intuitive sustenance scale is, for the most part, to depend on your impulses with respect to food decisions.

Guideline Two:

Respect Your Hunger
Keep your body organically encouraged with adequate vitality and sugars. Else you can bring about base travel to indulge. When you reach the top appetite, all aims of moderate, conscious eating are passing and unessential. Seeing how to respect this first organic sign units the phase for revamping trust with yourself and dinners.

While most diets need you to object to a growling stomach, intuitive nutrition renews your body's signals. You'll make sense of how to be increasingly aware of your food yearnings and how precisely to react appropriately to it before you feel hungry. Attempt this in the home: Before each dinner, rate your level of yearning, record a couple of internal signals that you saw, and enough time of day. Do this for week by week, and you'll are more in order together with your hunger, and furthermore which foods convey dependable vitality and the ones that are quickly catching fire and convey short-lived satiety.

Guideline Three:

MAKE PEACE WITH FOOD

Call a détente; quit the food battle! Give unconditional approval to food. In the event that you illuminate yourself that you can't or shouldn't have a particular food, it can bring about serious feelings of hardship that incorporate with wild longings and, regularly, gorging. At the point when you at last "give up" to your illegal foods, eating will be acquainted with such force, it, for the most part, results in Last Supper overeating and overpowering blame. Intuitive eating solicits that you forsake the idea from awful and the great food. That system energizes an unsafe 'win big or bust by any stretch of the imagination' attitude that may bring about longings for 'taboo' foods, joined by gorging and a rush of self-hatred and disgrace. Intuitive eating advances the hypothesis that food ought to be viewed as an actual existence upgrading experience.

Guideline Four:

Challenge The Meals Police
Shout a boisterous "basically no" to contemplations in your mind that proclaim you're "extraordinary" for eating under one thousand calories or "horrendous" in light of the fact that you ate a touch of chocolate cake. THE MEALS LAW AUTHORIZATIONS POLICE, the nonsensical rules that dieting has created. The police headquarters is certainly housed somewhere down in your mind, and its own amplifier yells ominous points, sad expressions, and blame inciting arraignments. Pursuing the suppers Police aside is a significant advance in time for Intuitive Eating. An escalated mental housekeeping and reframing disposition toward suppers are pivotal. Watch any food law authorization considerations you may have, such as "I was poor today" or "I shouldn't eat that." Resist the possibility that your food alternatives characterize it and the value it brings to the world. Pay special mind to people who might be deliberately or unwittingly showing a food police mindset, at that point talk about your intuitive eating way of

thinking with them and have them to help you by hushing up about their terrible remarks.

Guideline Five:

Feel Your Fullness
Tune in for the body flags that let you realize that you are not any hungrier. Pay heed to the signs that show that you're effectively full. Interruption in the focal point of suppers or nibble and have yourself the manner in which the food tastes, and what your present completion level is.

The other side of regarding your appetite is to regard when you're full. Since diet programs limit what, when, and exactly the amount you expend, it's easy to get detached from the internal signs that transmission satiety. At the point when you practice intuitive expending you take up a feast with a lesser degree of food yearnings and in a mentality which enables you to turn out to be increasingly fragile to prompts that you're full. In addition, you comprehend that you could refuel at whatever point you're ravenous once more, and you won't encounter constrained to clean your plate totally. Evaluate this at home: Make utilization of a satiety scale all through suppers to prepare your brain to address signs of satiety. Record perceptions of how you are feeling and all that you ate. This can help decide when to leave the fork and let the dinners actually feel supported and empowered.

Guideline Six:

Reveal The Satisfaction Factor
JAPAN has the knowledge to keep joy as you of their objectives of sound living. Inside our anger to be thin and sound, we regularly ignore likely the essential presents of presence the happiness and fulfilment, which can be inside the eating experience. At the point when you take in what you need, in a domain that is welcoming, the fulfilment you

infer is incredible power in helping you are feeling fulfilled and content. By giving this experience to yourself, you will see that it takes essentially less food to pick; you've had "enough."

Intuitive eating urges you to perceive foods that really cause you to feel great all through supper, yet a short time later, as well. You will find yourself floating towards and time for the foods that produce you feel your absolute best. Besides to relishing suppers and eating groceries that taste extraordinary and make you feel incredible, you can connect the entirety of your faculties: slow down, acknowledge what kind of food looks, regard how it achieved your plate, inhale every one of the fragrances, and eat inside a domain that appears to be acceptable expedite the plants and candles-and with people who light you up.

Guideline Seven:

Adapt Together To Your Emotions Without Needing Food
Discover approaches to solace and simplicity, sustain, occupy, and illuminate your passionate worries without utilizing food. Stress, depression, weariness, and outrage are sentiments a large portion of us experience all through presence. Everyone has its trigger, and every offer its own conciliation. Suppers won't fix these sentiments. It could comfort for the present moment, divert from the distress, or really numb you directly into a food aftereffect. However, food won't solve the problem. In the event that anything, eating for an enthusiastic yearning is just going to make you feel more awful after some time. You'll, in the end, need to adapt to the wellspring of the feeling, alongside the distress of overeating.

Indeed, food could be encouraging, yet that delight just keeps going insofar as the food. A short time later, anything that was eating you stays, covered under food, perhaps now offered with a piece of blame and disgrace. Intuitive eating urges you to perceive whether you're sense on edge, exhausted, desolate, tragic, or irate and look for a veritable arrangement. Get a walk, call a dear companion, practice reflection or yoga, get a remedial back rub, read a composed book, or make in a diary. You'll comprehend you're reacting appropriately when the reaction empowers you to feel good, not more terrible.

Guideline Eight:

Respect Your Body
Acknowledge your hereditary outline. Just for the most part in light of the fact that an individual with a footwear size of eight wouldn't ordinarily foresee reasonably to crush directly into a size six, it truly is correspondingly useless (and horrendous) to have a comparable desire regarding the matter of body size. Regard the body, so you can encounter

better about who you are. It's difficult to dismiss the dietary plan attitude in the event that you are ridiculous and excessively pivotal of the body shape.

Our varieties are our superpowers, but we live in a world that idealizes a cut body type. The possibility that individuals can profoundly change our life structures is typically unreasonable and ridiculous. Intuitive eating troubles you to grasp your hereditary plan set handy expectations, and praise your uniqueness. Evaluate this in the home: Anytime you catch yourself contrasting the body with someone else's, react as you'll if a buddy said something practically identical regarding themselves.

Guideline Nine:

Exercise-Feel The Difference
Disregard activist exercise. Just get dynamic and experience the distinction. Move your concentrate to how it appears to go your body, as opposed to the fat consuming limit impact of the activity. On the off chance that you focus on how you are feeling from working out, such as empowered, it could have the effect between turning up for an energetic morning hour's walk and striking the rest caution. If when you stirred, your solitary target is to lose abundance weight, rarely do you get an inspiring component at that time of period.

People who practice intuitive benefiting from appreciating practice since it gives them vitality improves their inclination, advances self-adequacy, and makes them experience solid, adaptable, and dexterous. Preparing isn't about which movement will consume off the most calories, however rather about which action might be the best time and stimulating. It's another exemplary instance of the manner in which the fulfilment factor could make propensities stick. The exercise you appreciate is an exercise that you're bound to do it once more, creating the force that drives feasible, long haul bliss.

Guideline Ten:

Respect Your Healthy And Soft Food
Choose foods that respect your prosperity and taste buds while making you feel better. Comprehend that you don't have to eat a perfect diet to be invigorating. You won't all of a sudden get yourself a supplement lack, or put on weight in one bite, one food, or one day of eating. It's what you normally eat after some time that issues. Progress, not so much flawlessness, is what makes a difference.

Recognizing how your prosperity impacts the wealth, you will ever have shallow known purposes behind health objectives and grounds your thought processes in what is important: your individual qualities. Getting the point of view on why health is significant can assist you with the understanding that no supper or chomp could represent the moment of truth your self-esteem. Adjust your prosperity to your aspirations, and you will be significantly progressively inspired to develop rehearses that help your day by day life objectives.

AN ACTIVITY WITH GREAT REWARDS
Numerous people have been disappointed with their association with food and their bodies. Many experienced endeavoured either formal or casual dieting and had encountered disappointment and gloom. By learning the ideas of Intuitive Consuming and putting them to work, many will find an extending of the evaluation of life and quality about eating. You can go as well!

Chapter 9: Arousing the Intuitive Eater: Stages

The journey to Intuitive Eating is like going for a cross-district climbing trip. Before you really tie without anyone else climbing boots, you'd have to recognize what's in store all through your outing. While a road map is viable, it doesn't disclose what you'll be enough prepared, such as trail conditions, atmosphere, special touring detects, the kind of garments to put on, etc. The goal of this part is, for the most part, to help you comprehend what to envision all through your outing to Intuitive Eating.

Regardless of whether it's strolling or relearning an unmistakably all the more fulfilling eating plan, you will continue through numerous phases in transit. The amount of time that you should remain static in a specific stage is certainly a factor and amazingly individualized. For example, crossing new climbing trails relies on how physically fit you are, the way you adapt to worry with a new path, exactly how much time you have to climb, and the choice of climbing trails. In like manner, your adventure back again to Intuitive Eating relies on how protracted you've been dieting, how emphatically settled in your everyday diet believing is the means by which long you've been utilizing suppers to deal with life, that you are so arranged to confide in yourself, and that you are so prepared to put weight decrease on the storage compartment burner and see how to turn into an Intuitive Eater the essential objective.

Now and again, you'll move in reverse and advances among the stages. In the event that you recognize that is an ordinary segment of the procedure, it can assist you with continuing without inclination that you will fall away from the faith or not so much gaining ground.

Think about this circumstance: You are on a mobile path and experience a fork in the road that is difficult to unravel together with your path map. Do you go legitimately to one side or left? You consider for quite a while and pick to go remaining. While strolling, you place something you've in no way, shape or form seen previously, a sparkling green caterpillar shimmying up a purple bloom. A couple of activities ahead, you find a novel fowl. In any case, a couple of strategies past these wonders of character are a huge rock flagging that you locate an inappropriate course. You pivot, return to the fork, and think about the other course. Was this temporary re-routing an exercise in futility?

No! So also, in connection to Intuitive Eating, you will require numerous turns and test out new contemplations and practices. You may locate that subsequent to creating recognizable advancement, and you return to old procedures are terrible and unfulfilling. In any case, such as gaining "an inappropriate" course on the grand trekking trail, you'll see that outings into matured expending examples can be used as learning encounters. (Numerous climbers wouldn't ordinarily scold themselves to be uncertain of what direction to take; rather, they'd be grateful for the disclosures of character that a blocked course offered.) It's imperative that you help yourself out and welcome the preparation that turns out from experience. This procedure includes originating from a position of interest rather than a position of judgment, along these lines whatever you do; don't crush yourself up intellectually!

Intuitive Eating is very not equivalent to dieting. Dieters, for the most part, get disappointed on the off chance that they don't follow the dietary plan way decisively as endorsed. We've seen numerous a relentless dieters simply have an off-base change at one feast, be critical for that error, and "blow" the dietary plan for that day time or end of the week or in reality longer! Recall that the outing to Intuitive Eating is typically a procedure, loaded up with good and bad times, un-like dieting where in actuality the regular desire is unquestionably direct advancement (losing a specific measure of abundance weight in a specific time span).

The road to Intuitive Eating is like obtaining a long haul common store. Over the long haul, you will see an arrival on speculation, paying little mind to the everyday vacillations of the money markets. It is customary and anticipated. How amusing that individuals have been prepared that, in financial matters, the everyday changes in the cash markets are typical, and once in a while is there a moment get-rich fix, yet, in the multibillion-dollar, a year pounds misfortune business, "get slender quick" might be the main target for accomplishment. We are contributed, rather, in helping you give harmony to your expending presence and self-perception. In connection to this objective, remember Webster's portrayal of procedure: "a continuous advancement including numerous alterations" and "a particular way to deal with accomplishing something, including various advances or activities by and large."

Much like any procedure, it's essential that you remain centred in, and develop from the numerous experiences you will experience. Assuming, in any case, you focus on the result (which for some, people is fat or the number of pounds lost), it could make you experience overpowered and debilitated, and wrap up disrupting the strategy. Rather, if your air conditioning information little changes in transit and worth the preparation encounters (that may in some cases be disappointing), it can assist you with adhering to the Intuitive Eating course and push ahead. When you truly become an Intuitive Eater, you will consistently check out your inward insight, and you may feel better on a basic level, body, and soul.

Now, we feel it is important to explain the issue of the mission for weight reduction. For a few, the body will return to its normal abundance weight level, which might be not exactly your present pounds and remain there. To watch if this relates to you, ask yourself the following inquiries: Perhaps you have routinely destroyed from agreeable totality level? Perform you routinely gorge when you're getting arranged for the following diet (understanding that there will turn into a ton of foods you won't be allowed to eat on the dietary plan)? Perform your gorge as an adapting framework in troublesome events or to fill period when you're exhausted? Maybe you have been impervious to work out?

Do you only exercise in the event that you are dieting? Do you skip foods or hold back to eat until you're insatiably hungry, possibly to find that you indulge when you at long last expend? Do you are feeling remorseful; either when you indulge or when you take in all that you call a "poor food," which results in all the more overeating? If you addressed "yes" for a few of the vast majority of these inquiries, after that all things considered, your present weight might be more prominent than the weight the body is intended to keep up. Furthermore, it is likely you will have the option to return to your common, sound weight, because of this procedure. Be that as it may, recall, weight decrease should be put on the storage compartment burner. In the event that you focus on weight reduction, it'll meddle with your ability to settle on decisions predicated on your intuitive signs.

When you've surrendered the pointlessness of dieting perpetually, you'll wind up eating far fewer suppers with a craving to see customary movement in your day by day life. You'll find that the body feels so far superior when your midsection isn't stuffed, at whatever point your muscle tissue is conditioned, just as your heart is coordinate. You will likewise find that as your contemplations about your eating and body begin to transform, you will encounter an all the more loosening up feeling, rather than the incessant foundation stress that weaving machines each supper decision. Nonetheless, if you keep on focusing on weight decrease as the objective, you'll get tangled up in the matured diet-attitude figuring, which won't serve you.

Throughout the years, we've seen our people continue through a five-organize movement in figuring out how to be an Intuitive Eater. The following segment can assist you with getting an idea of what things to expect inside your very own adventure.

Stage One: Readiness-Hitting Diet Plan Bottom
This is the place numerous individuals start. You are agonizingly conscious that each attempt to get in shape is made in "falling flat." You are wary of esteeming every day predicated on whether the level is as a rule up or down a pound or two (or on the off chance that you indulged your prior day). You envision and stress over dinners constantly. You talk the prohibitive food visit "Just in the event that I didn't have to watch my overabundance weight, I could expend that," or "I encountered two treats I truly was awful today."

As of now, your weight might be higher than any time in recent memory, or, without significantly over-weight, you lose and increase five or ten pounds to such an extent and rapidly as you wash your garments in addition to they get filthy again! You have lost contact with organic food longings and satiety signals.

You have overlooked all that you truly prefer to expend and rather eat all that you figure you "should" eat. Your association with dinners has built up a poor tone, and you fear to eat the foods you like since you're apprehensive it'll be difficult to stop. At the point when you yield to the enticement of illegal foods, it's normal to indulge them, since you are feeling remorseful. However, you earnestly pledge you won't ever eat them again.

It's not bizarre to get that you take into comfort, occupy, or even numb yourself from your very own emotions. On the off chance that that is the situation, you will feel that an incredible evaluation offers been blurred by obsession thinking about suppers and by careless expending.

The self-perception is negative-you don't simply like the manner in which you show up and feel inside your body, and confidence is reduced. You have found from your experience that dieting won't work-you have arrived in a desperate predicament and experience stuck, debilitated, and disheartened.

This stage proceeds until you select that you will be troubled eating and living along these lines you will be prepared to accomplish something positive about it. Your first contemplations may veer toward finding another diet to determine your issues. Yet, very quickly, you comprehend that you can't do that one until kingdom come. On the off chance that that is the place you find yourself, you at that point are set up for the method that will empower you to get back again to eating intuitively.

Stage Two: Exploration-Conscious Learning And Quest For Pleasure
That is a phase of investigation and disclosure. You will continue through a phase of hyper consciousness to incredibly help reacquaint yourself together with your intuitive signs: hunger, season inclinations, and satiety.

This stage resembles figuring out how precisely to drive a vehicle. For the beginner driver, simply getting the vehicle out from the garage requires a lot of conscious deduction, loaded up with a psychological agenda: Place the principle component in the start, make certain the contraption is in diversion zone or impartial, start the motor, check the rearview reflect, remove the hand brake, and so forth. This hyper consciousness is basic to secure every one of the means required simply to acquire that vehicle into Drive! In a similar inclination, you will focus in on subtleties of eating which have advanced without such centred reasoning. (In any case, this is basic to recover the Intuitive Eater in you.)

It might seem clumsy and awkward, fanatical even. In any case, hyper consciousness varies than over the top considering. Over the top reasoning is generally unavoidable and is viewed as stress. It fills your brain during most of the day and prevents you from considering much else. Hyperconsciousness is increasingly specific. It zooms in the event that you have thought about food, yet leaves totally when the eating experience is finished. What's more, like the means required stresses become autopilot for the accomplished driver, Intuitive Eating will eventually get experienced without this fundamental ungainliness.

You may accept that you are in a hyperconscious state more often than not during this stage. This may feel awkward at first just as maybe even abnormal. Keep in mind, a ton of your prior eating was either primarily thoughtless or diet plan coordinated.

In this stage, you'll begin to make harmony with food giving yourself unqualified consent to expend. This part may feel frightening, and you may choose to move gradually (inside your solace level). Become acquainted with to wipe out blame incited eating and begin to find the requirement for the fulfilment component with food. The significantly progressively cheerful you are while expending, the substantially less you see food on the off chance that you are not hungry you won't wind up being lurking here and there.

You will explore different avenues regarding foods that you probably won't have eaten for quite a while. This comprises of sifting through your exact food needs and needs. You may even find that you don't simply like the kind of a couple of the foods you've been longing for! (Remember those long stretches of dieting, or eating all that you "should" simply serve to disengage you from your own inner eating travel and genuine food decisions.) Become acquainted with to respect your food yearnings and perceive the body markers that show the innumerable degrees of appetite. Become acquainted with, to separate these organic pointers from the enthusiastic markers that may likewise trigger eating.

In this stage, you may find that you will eat bigger degrees of foods than the body needs. It will be difficult to regard your totality as of now since you will require time to try out the amount it requires to satisfy a denied sense of taste. What's more, it requires some serious energy that you ought to create trust with suppers again and comprehend that it's really okay to expend. By what means will you respect completion, on the off chance that you are not absolutely sure it's okay to eat the specific food, or if you fear it won't become there tomorrow?

In the event that you have recently been putting on overabundance weight, weight gain typically stops or is restricted to just a couple of pounds. At the point when you have been utilizing suppers inwardly, you may find that you will begin to feel your emotions and may encounter uneasiness, pity, or really sadness on occasion.

Most of your eating could be foods that are heavier in fat and sugar than you've been familiar with in spite of the fact that you may have been eating huge degrees of these food types furtively or with blame. How you eat in this stage will never be the example that you'll set up or requirement for a lifetime. You will see that your nourishing soundness is for the most part helter-skelter and you probably won't feel physically alongside focuses during this time. That is all standard and anticipated. You have to let yourself continue through this phase for such a long time as you need. Keep in mind, and you are creating for quite a while of hardship, troublesome self-talk, and blame. You are re-building positive food experiences, much the same as a strand of pearls. Every feast experience, similar to each pearl, may seem immaterial, however, by and large, they change lives.

Stage Three: Crystallization
In this stage, you will experience the primary renewals of the Intuitive Eating style which has consistently been a piece of you, yet was covered underneath the flotsam and jetsam of dieting. At the point when you enter this stage, a great deal of the investigation work from the earlier stage begins to solidify and feels as if strong conducts change. Your thoughts regarding food are not any more over the top. You barely need to stay aware of the hyperconsciousness about eating that was initially required. Thusly, your eating choices don't require very as particularly coordinated accepted. Rather, you find that your food choices and reactions to natural pointers are principally intuitive.

You have a bigger feeling of trust-both in your to pick what you really need to eat and in the undeniable reality that your natural signs are depend-capable. You are advantageous with your food choices and will start to see expanded satisfaction at your suppers.

Now, you respect your appetite most of the time and it's less difficult to perceive what you feel simply like eating in the event that you are hungry. You keep on creating harmony with food.

What feels new in this stage is that it's more straightforward to require some investment out in the midst of your food to intentionally check exactly how a lot of your paunch is topping off. It is conceivable to watch your completion and regard the presence of that sign, regardless of whether you find that you as often as possible eat past the totality tag. Precisely like when a toxophilite requires focus on a crisp objective, it frequently requires catching numerous bolts before figuring out how precisely to come to the bull's-eye. You may at present be picking recently prohibited foods most of the time, yet you will find that you don't require as a lot of them to satisfy you.

On the off chance that you've been a genuinely signaled eater, you'll become very skilled at isolating natural yearning markers from passionate appetite. Because of this lucidity, more than not frequently, you'll be encountering your feelings and discovering techniques to com-stronghold and occupy yourself without the use of food.

Be certain you put weight decrease on the storage compartment burner. Much more significant than abundance weight reduction, is the inclination of well-turning out to be and strengthening that become-gins to happen. You won't any longer feel vulnerable and miserable. You will begin to regard your body and get that in case you're over your regular weight, it's because of the dieting attitude, rather than absence of resolve.

Stage 4: The Intuitive Eater Awakens

By enough time you arrive at this stage, all the work you have just been doing comes full circle in an agreeable, free-streaming eating style. You consistently pick what you truly need to eat when you are ravenous. Since you comprehend that you can have altogether more suppers, based on your personal preference, when you are starving, it's anything but difficult to stop eating when you are feeling serenely full.

You may begin to find that you pick more advantageous foods, not on the grounds that you envision you should, but since you are feeling better physically when you take along these lines. The pressing need to demonstrate to yourself that you could have recently prohibited foods could have reduced. You truly know and trust these foods will be there, and on the off chance that you need to eat them truly, you can-in this manner they drop their charming quality. Chocolate starts to shield myself against a similar mental implication as a peach. You won't any more drawn out need to test yourself, just as your hardship reaction with suppers will be no more.

At the point when you do choose the foods you used to limit, you'll get extraordinary delight, and feel content with a particularly littler amount than beforehand, and without blame. (At the point when you are feeling regretful eating a suppers, it removes a great deal of the happiness from eating.)

In the event that managing your emotions have been hard for you, you'll be less reluctant to see them, and be increasingly capable at plunking down with them. Finding refreshing choices to occupy and comfort yourself when required can be normal for you.

Your food talk and self talk will be certain and non-basic. Your tranquility settlement with suppers is solidly settled, and you will have discharged any contention or remaining blame about dinner's decisions you have hauled around.

You have quit being furious together with your body and making ill bred input about it. You regard it and acknowledge there are a wide range of shapes and sizes on the planet. At this genuine point, and if it's intended to be, the body will be coming to moving toward its natural weight.

Stage Five: The Ultimate Stage-Treasure The Pleasure

Right now your Intuitive Eater has been guaranteed. You will confide in your body's intuitive capacities it will be easy to respect your yearning and regard totality. At long last, you will encounter no blame about your feast decisions or amounts. Since you like your sentimental relationship to dinners and fortune the fulfillment that eating currently offers you, you will dispose of unacceptable eating conditions and unappealing foods.

You should encounter benefiting from in the most ideal of conditions as opposed to corrupt it with enthusiastic misery. You will encounter an internal conviction to quit utilizing food to deal with enthusiastic circumstances, if that is your propensity. At the point when sentiments become too astounding, you will see that you'll much rather adapt to your feelings or occupy yourself at times from their site with anything separated from food.

Since your eating style has become a wellspring of joy rather than a suffering, you will encounter sustenance and development in various manners.

The duty of activity will be evacuated, and practicing will begin to look luring to you. Exercise won't be used as a driving strain to catch fire more calories; rather, you feel com-mitted to exercise with an end goal to feel much improved, and intellectually physically. In like manner, food won't be another instrument to make you feel terrible about how you eat; rather, it transforms into an approach to feeling as in reality great and solid as could be expected under the circumstances.

At the point when you arrive at a definitive stage, your bodyweight will sink into what's normal for you-a spot that is agreeable and befitting your height and body outline. In the event that your bodyweight was at that point ordinary, you will find that you'll keep up it without exertion and you will be freed of the mental good and bad times that go with the confinement/overeating cycles.

Finally, you will encounter enabled and shielded from outside powers telling you what and exactly the amount to eat, and how the body should look. You will feel clear of the duty of dieting. What's more, you'll be an Intuitive Eater again.

That you can do it!
These stages and the progressions that happen with your eating and considerations may seem outlandish. Or on the other hand, it may show up excessively startling. For instance, the very idea of giving yourself unrestricted authorization to eat may seem unnerving and you may expect that you'll never stop eating or putting on abundance weight. The remainder of the distribution clarifies in extraordinary fine detail how precisely to execute every rule, why it truly is required, and the explanation behind it. Also, you will figure out how extra interminable dieters became Intuitive Eaters and how it changed their lives. By enough time you wrap up this book, you will unquestionably realize that you also may turn into an Intuitive Eater, and forestall the franticness of dieting.

Conclusion

Thank you for reading this book!

Now you have all the instructions to perform Atkins Diet in the best possible way!

EMOTIONAL EATING

Break the Cycle, Say STOP Binge Eating! A Proven 21-Day Program Based on Ten Intuitive Principles for a Healthy Relationship with Food. Be Free from the Slavery of Hunger (Part 1)

By
Kelly Francis

© Copyright 2020 - All rights reserved.

The content contained within this book may not be reproduced, duplicated or transmitted without direct written permission from the author or the publisher.

Under no circumstances will any blame or legal responsibility be held against the publisher, or author, for any damages, reparation, or monetary loss due to the information contained within this book. Either directly or indirectly.

Legal Notice:

This book is copyright protected. This book is only for personal use. You cannot amend, distribute, sell, use, quote or paraphrase any part, or the content within this book, without the consent of the author or publisher.

Disclaimer Notice:

Please note the information contained within this document is for educational and entertainment purposes only. All effort has been executed to present accurate, up to date, and reliable, complete information. No warranties of any kind are declared or implied. Readers acknowledge that the author is not engaging in the rendering of legal, financial, medical or professional advice. The content within this book has been derived from various sources. Please consult a licensed professional before attempting any techniques outlined in this book.

By reading this document, the reader agrees that under no circumstances is the author responsible for any losses, direct or indirect, which are incurred as a result of the use of information contained within this document, including, but not limited to, — errors, omissions, or inaccuracies.

INTRODUCTION

Emotional Eating: Break the Cycle, Say STOP Binge Eating! A Proven-Effective 21-Day Program Based On Ten Intuitive Principles For A Healthy Relationship With Food. Find Freedom From Dieting Forever. Emotional eating is described as "the urge to eat in reaction to positive and negative feelings." While the word emotional eating mostly applies to eating as a means of coping with negative emotions, it also includes eating for positive emotions, such as eating food while enjoying an accomplishment or eating to boost an already good mood. Emotions often guide the feeding in these conditions but not in a negative way.

Any people get to terms with difficult situations by having comfort food. Chowing on ice cream or macaroni, and cheese will make it look like it's all right. And maybe there is an explanation why.

As points out, parts of the brain are punished with eating high-fat or high-sugar items. And more than a decade of psychological research shows that any rewarding activity would possibly replicate itself.

Emotional feeding means eating for purposes other than hunger. You can eat for being unhappy, upset, tired or lonely. Or you could be using food as a reward. Nutrition will find you relaxing and divert you from what really does concern you.

Eating comfort food as things get tough — also recognized as emotional eating or eating stress — is not, though, an answer to the challenges of life. It only works briefly. Worse, if it brings on weight gain, it creates longer-term anxiety.

Knowing what causes your emotional eating: Another way to control emotional eating is to find out what the symptoms are. Keep a food diary that not only tracks what you eat and how much but also how you felt at the time.

When you identify a trend, build a turnaround plan. For starters, if you often eat because you believe after a bad day you deserve it, realize that you also deserve to lose weight, feel healthy and be proud of yourself. If you are eating because of tension, learn to turn the discomfort down. Yoga, meditation and regular exercise may help to lower levels of stress.

Reasons of emotional eating: When finding out why you need comfort food you may be able to stop panic eating or emotional eating. Is it calming you down, cheering you up, making up for a bad day or a combination? Recognizing such patterns of thought can promote resistance to giving in. It also helps to understand that emotional eating is not solving the problem that led you to get angry.

The greatest breaks from emotional eating are activities that only require about five minutes switching gears— just long enough to help.

Several suggestions for moving strategies include: walking outside for a five-minute walk, turning on your favorite music and dancing, contacting a close friend to talk. The more ways you will think about entertaining yourself, the better it will become to stop eating tension over time. Instead it will become your new habit of fighting.

If you're an emotional eater, you may not notice the inherent signs of appetite and fullness in your body. You should eat more than you need or wish for.Emotional eating may interfere with making healthy choices regarding food. And it can keep you from getting to and remaining at a healthy weight.

What are symptoms of mental sustenance?

Everybody feeds from time to time, for purposes other than thirst. But if you find that out of hunger or for relaxation you sometimes search for food, you may be consuming for emotional reasons.

Common signs of emotional eating are: if you have more stress in your life, adjust your eating habits.
Feed if you're not thirsty, or are full.
Eating to soothe feelings.
Meat is used as a compliment.
Eating so as not to contend with a stressful situation.

Identify the emotional eating symptoms

One way to find out what emotional eating causes is to keep a diary of food. Factor in when and what you're doing. Write down also what you do and felt before you started eating. To find patterns in your eating habits, you can use this knowledge. For starters, you might find that you purchase an unhealthy snack from the office vending machine any time you start thinking about an assignment at work.

Use a scale of hunger: A scale of hunger will help you learn how to tell the difference between real, actual hunger and hunger in your mind. Psychological appetite is an eating impulse triggered by feelings, such as pain, anxiety, disappointment, or joy.

Value your appetite on a scale of 1 to 10 as you start feeling like you want something to eat, with 1 starving and 10 being so loaded you feel sick. A 5 or 6 rating means that you're comfortable— neither too hungry nor too whole.

Emotional eating is a form of reducing or relaxing negative emotions, such as tension, rage, anxiety, depression, sorrow and loneliness. Major events in life or, more generally, the daily life hassles may cause negative emotions that contribute to emotional eating and hinder the attempts to lose weight.

1—Starving, exhausted, dizzy 2—Very thin, cranky, low-energy, plenty of stomach rumbling 3—Pretty tired, stomach rumbling a little 4—Starting to feel a little better 5—Satisfied, neither hungry nor complete 6—A little full, comfortably full 7—A little awkward 8—Feeling bloated 9—Very cramped, stomach hurts 10—So loaded you feel sick Use the scale to evaluate your appetite. If you feel like eating but your degree of hunger is a scale 6 or higher, pause and test your emotions.

Unpleasant eating happens when the diet becomes the reaction of an individual to certain unpleasant internal or external signals. The emotional eater may consume comfort foods rather than dealing in their thoughts and the stress they put in in an effort to distract themselves from the pain. This also includes, in most situations, a form of compulsive overeating that results in an overly full stomach sensation. Of reality, consuming this sort of food does not come without negative side effects. Three of the most famous are in the order.

Weight-related health concerns: Depression, high blood pressure, exhaustion and high cholesterol are all health issues that may come from frequent emotional eating outbursts.

Guilt: They're usually filled with guilt and shame for what they've done after the emotional "threat" has passed and the emotional

overeater has eaten up. This guilt may contribute to another episode of emotional eating or low self-esteem.

Diarrhea: As nervous eaters often over-eat or eat too fast and suffer stomach pain or diarrhea afterwards, because the sight of food in the stomach acts as a diversion to the feelings they are trying to avoid. It can last a day or two after the actual meal.

We don't forever eat simply to satisfy physical hunger. several folks conjointly communicate food for comfort, stress relief, or to reward ourselves. And after we do, we tend to tend to succeed in for food, sweets, and different comforting however unhealthy foods. you may reach for a pint of frozen dessert once you're feeling down, order a pizza pie if you're bored or lonely, or swing by the drive-through once a nerve-wracking day at work. Emotional feeding is exploitation food to form yourself feel better—to fill emotional desires, instead of your abdomen. sadly, emotional feeding doesn't fix emotional issues. In fact, it always causes you to feel worse. Afterward, not solely will the first emotional issue stay, however you furthermore mght feel guilty for mortal sin.

People who showing emotion eat reach for food many times every week or a lot of to suppress and soothe negative feelings. they will even feel guilt or shame once feeding this manner, resulting in a cycle of excess feeding and associated problems, like weight gain.

The emotional feeding cycle
Occasionally exploitation food as a pick-me-up, a reward, or to celebrate isn't essentially a nasty factor. however once feeding is your primary emotional header mechanism—when your 1st impulse is to open the white goods whenever you're stressed, upset, angry, lonely, exhausted, or bored—you grind to a halt in an unhealthy cycle wherever the important feeling or drawback is rarely addressed.

Emotional hunger can't be crammed with food. feeding could feel sensible within the moment, however the sentiments that triggered the feeding are still there. And you regularly feel worse than you probably did before owing to the uncalled-for calories you've simply consumed. You beat yourself for messing up and not having a lot of resolution.

Compounding the matter, you stop learning healthier ways in which to upset your emotions, you've got a more durable and harder time dominant your weight, and you are feeling more and more overcome over each food and your feelings. however in spite of however overcome you are feeling over food and your feelings, it's potential to form a positive amendment. you'll be able to learn healthier ways in which to upset your emotions, avoid triggers, conquer cravings, and at last place a stop to emotional feeding.

The distinction between emotional hunger and physical hunger

Before you'll be able to become independent from from the cycle of emotional feeding, you initially got to learn the way to differentiate between emotional and physical hunger. this will be trickier than it sounds, particularly if you frequently use food to upset your feelings.

Emotional hunger will be powerful, thus it's simple to mistake it for physical hunger. however there are clues you'll be able to seek for to assist you tell physical and emotional hunger apart.

Emotional hunger comes on suddenly. It hits you in an immediate and feels overwhelming and pressing. Physical hunger, on the opposite hand, comes on a lot of bit by bit. The urge to eat doesn't feel as dire or demand instant satisfaction (unless you haven't ingested for a awfully long time).

Emotional hunger craves specific comfort foods. once you're physically hungry, nearly something sounds good—including healthy stuff like vegetables. however emotional hunger craves food or sugar-coated snacks that offer an immediate rush. you are feeling such as you would like cheesecake or pizza pie, and zilch else can do.

Emotional hunger usually results in mindless feeding. Before you recognize it, you've ingested an entire bag of chips or an entire pint of frozen dessert while not extremely listening or totally enjoying it. once you're feeding in response to physical hunger, you're usually a lot of awake to what you're doing.

Emotional hunger isn't glad once you're full. you retain wanting a lot of and more, usually feeding till you're uncomfortably stuffed. Physical hunger, on the opposite hand, doesn't got to be stuffed. you are feeling glad once your abdomen is full.

Emotional hunger isn't set within the abdomen. instead of a growling belly or a pang in your abdomen, you are feeling your hunger as a desire you can't get out of your head. You're targeted on specific textures, tastes, and smells.

Emotional hunger usually results in regret, guilt, or shame. after you eat to satisfy physical hunger, you're unlikely to feel guilty or mortified as a result of you're merely giving your body what it desires. If you are feeling guilty once you eat, it's probably as a result of you recognize at bottom that you're not feeding for organic process reasons.

Emotional hunger vs. Physical hunger

Emotional hunger comes on suddenly Physical hunger comes on bit by bit

Emotional hunger looks like it must be glad instantly Physical hunger will wait

Emotional hunger craves specific comfort foods Physical hunger is receptive options—lots of things sound sensible

Emotional hunger isn't glad with a full abdomen. Physical hunger stops once you're full

Emotional feeding triggers feelings of guilt, quality, and shame feeding to satisfy physical hunger doesn't cause you to feel dangerous regarding yourself

Identify your emotional feeding triggers

The first step in putt a stop to emotional feeding is distinctive your personal triggers. What things, places, or feelings cause you to reach for the comfort of food? Most emotional feeding is coupled to unpleasant feelings, however it may be triggered by positive emotions, like appreciated yourself for achieving a goal or celebrating a vacation or blessed event.

CHAPTER 1:

Common causes of emotional feeding

Stress – Ever notice however stress causes you to hungry? It's not simply in your mind. once stress is chronic, because it thus usually is in our chaotic, fast world, your body produces high levels of the strain secretion, cortisol. corticoid triggers cravings for salty, sweet, and deep-fried foods—foods that provide you with a burst of energy and pleasure. The a lot of uncontrolled stress in your life, the a lot of probably you're to show to food for emotional relief.

Stuffing emotions – feeding will be the way to briefly silence or "stuff down" uncomfortable emotions, as well as anger, fear, sadness, anxiety, loneliness, resentment, and shame. whereas you're desensitising yourself with food, you'll be able to avoid the tough emotions you'd rather not feel.

Boredom or feelings of emptiness – does one ever eat merely to offer yourself one thing to try to to, to alleviate tedium, or as the way to fill a void in your life? you are feeling unrealized and empty, and food could be a thanks to occupy your mouth and it slow. within the moment, it fills you up and distracts you from underlying feelings of aimlessness and discontentment together with your life.

Childhood habits – remember to your childhood recollections of food. Did your oldsters reward sensible behavior with frozen dessert, take you out for pizza pie after you got an honest information, or serve you sweets after you were feeling sad? These habits will usually carry over into adulthood. Or your feeding is also driven by nostalgia—for cherished recollections of cooking burgers within the curtilage together with your pappa or baking and eating cookies with your female parent.

Social influences – obtaining along with others for a meal could be a good way to alleviate stress, however it may cause mortal sin. It's simple to satiate just because the food is there or because everybody else is feeding. you will conjointly satiate in social things out of nervousness. Or maybe your family or circle of friends encourages you to satiate, and it's easier to travel in conjunction with the cluster.

Keep an emotional feeding diary

You probably recognized yourself in a minimum of some of the previous descriptions. however nevertheless, you'll wish to urge even a lot of specific. one in all the simplest ways in which to spot the patterns behind your emotional feeding is to stay track with a food and mood diary.

Every time you satiate or feel compelled to succeed in for your version of food Kryptonite, take an instant to work out what triggered the urge. If you turn back, you'll typically realize associate displeasing event that kicked of the emotional feeding cycle. Write it all down in your food and mood diary: what you Greek deity (or wished to eat), what happened to upset you, however you felt before you Greek deity, what you felt as you were feeding, and the way you felt later on.

Over time, you'll see a pattern emerge. perhaps you usually find yourself gorging yourself once outlay time with a essential friend. Or maybe you stress eat whenever you're on a point or after you attend family functions. Once you determine your emotional feeding triggers, succeeding step is distinctive healthier ways in which to feed your feelings.

Find different ways in which to feed your feelings

If you don't shrewdness to manage your emotions in a very manner that doesn't involve food, you won't be able to management your feeding habits for terribly long. Diets thus usually fail as a result of they provide logical organic process recommendation that solely works if you've got aware management over your feeding habits. It doesn't work once emotions hijack the method, exigent an instantaneous payoff with food.

In order to prevent emotional feeding, you've got to search out different ways in which to satisfy yourself showing emotion. It's not enough to know the cycle of emotional feeding or perhaps to understand your triggers, though that's an enormous opening move. you would like alternatives to food that you just will communicate for emotional fulfillment.

CHAPTER 2:

Alternatives to emotional feeding

I f you're depressed or lonely, decision somebody who forever causes you to feel higher, play together with your dog or cat, or check up on a favourite pic or cherished souvenir.

If you're anxious, expend your nervous energy by performing arts to your favorite song, compressing a stress ball, or taking a brisk walk.

If you're exhausted, treat yourself with a hot cup of tea, take a shower, lightweight some scented candles, or wrap yourself in a very heat blanket.

If you're bored, scan an honest book, watch a comedy show, explore the outside, or communicate associate activity you get pleasure from (woodworking, taking part in the stringed instrument, shooting hoops, scrapbooking, etc.).

Pause once cravings hit and sign on with yourself

Most emotional eaters feel overcome over their food cravings. once the urge to eat hits, it's all you'll be able to have confidence. you are feeling associate nearly unendurable tension that demands to be fed, right now! as a result of you've tried to resist within the past and unsuccessful, you think that your resolution simply isn't up to snuff. however the reality is that you just have a lot of power over your cravings than you're thinking that.

Take five before you throw in the towel to a desire

Emotional feeding tends to be automatic and nearly mindless. Before you even understand what you're doing, you've reached for a bath of frozen dessert and polished off 1/2 it. however if you'll be able to take an instant to pause and mirror once you're hit with a desire, you offer yourself the chance to form a distinct call.

Can you suspend feeding for 5 minutes? or simply begin with one minute. Don't tell yourself you can't throw in the towel to the craving; bear in mind, the taboo is very tempting. simply tell yourself to attend.

While you're waiting, sign on with yourself. however are you feeling? What's occurring emotionally? albeit you finish up feeding, you'll have an improved understanding of why you probably did it. this will assist you set yourself up for a distinct response next time.

Learn to simply accept your feelings—even the dangerous ones
While it should appear that the core drawback is that you're overcome over food, emotional feeding really stems from feeling overcome over your emotions. You don't feel capable of addressing your feelings head on, thus you avoid them with food.

Allowing yourself to feel uncomfortable emotions will be chilling. you will concern that, like Pandora's box, once you open the door you won't be able to shut it. however the reality is that after we don't obsess over or suppress our emotions, even the foremost painful and tough feelings subside comparatively quickly and lose their power to manage our attention.

To do this you would like to become conscious and learn the way to remain connected to your moment-to-moment emotional expertise. this will modify you to rein in stress and repair emotional issues that always trigger emotional feeding. HelpGuide's free Emotional Intelligence Toolkit will show you ways.

Indulge while not mortal sin by degustation your food
When you eat to feed your feelings, you tend to try to to thus quickly, senselessly intense food on autopilot. You eat thus quick you miss out on the various tastes and textures of your food—as well as your body's cues that you're full and not hungry. however by retardation down and degustation each bite, you'll not solely get pleasure from your food a lot of however you'll even be less probably to satiate.

Slowing down and degustation your food is a very important facet of conscious eating, the alternative of mindless, emotional feeding. attempt taking some deep breaths before beginning your food, putt your utensils down between bites, and extremely specializing in the expertise of feeding. listen to the textures, shapes, colours and smells of your food. however will every mouthful taste? however does it create your body feel? By retardation down during this manner, you'll realize you appreciate every bite of food way more. you'll be able to even fancy your favorite foods and feel full on a lot of less. It takes time for the body's fullness signal to succeed in your brain, thus taking some moments to contemplate however you are feeling once every bite—hungry or satiated—can assist you avoid mortal sin.

Practice conscious feeding
Eating whereas you're conjointly doing different things—such as looking TV, driving, or fidgeting with your phone—can forestall you from totally enjoying your food. Since your mind is elsewhere, you will not feel glad or continue feeding even supposing you're not hungry. feeding a lot of heedfully will facilitate focus your mind on your food and therefore the pleasure of a meal and curb mortal sin. See conscious feeding.

Support yourself with healthy life-style habits
When you're physically robust, relaxed, and well reinvigorated, you're higher able to handle the curveballs that life inevitably throws your manner. however once you're already exhausted and flooded, any very little hiccup has the potential to send you off the rails and straight toward the white goods. Exercise, sleep, and different healthy life-style habits can assist you get through tough times while not emotional feeding.

Make daily exercise a priority. Physical activity will wonders for your mood and energy levels, and it's conjointly a robust stress reducer. And moving into the exercise habit sophisticated} than you will assume.

Aim for eight hours of sleep nightly. after you don't get the sleep you would like, your body craves sugar-coated foods that may provide you with a fast energy boost. obtaining lots of rest can facilitate with appetency management and scale back food cravings.

Make time for relaxation.Give yourself permission to require a minimum of half-hour a day to relax, decompress, and unwind. this is often it slow to require a prospect from your responsibilities and recharge your batteries.

Connect with others. Don't underestimate the importance of shut relationships and social activities. outlay time with positive those who enhance your life can facilitate defend you from the negative effects of stress.

What causes somebody to eat owing to their emotions?

Anything from work stress to money worries, health problems to relationship struggles is also the basis cause of your emotional feeding.

It's a problem that affects each sexes. however in keeping with completely different studies, emotional feeding is a lot of common with ladies than with men.

Why food?
Negative emotions could cause a sense of emptiness or associate emotional void. Food is believed to be the way to fill that void and make a false feeling of "fullness" or temporary wholeness.

Other factors include:
retreating from social support throughout times of emotional would like not partaking in activities which may otherwise relieve stress, sadness, and so on not understanding the distinction between physical and emotional hunger using negative self-talking that's associated with bingeing episodes. this will produce a cycle of emotional feeding changing corticoid levels in response to worry, resulting in cravings.

Emotional feeding affects each men and girls. it should be caused by variety of things, as well as stress, secretion changes, or mixed hunger cues.
Physical hunger vs Emotional hunger
It develops slowly over time. It comes regarding suddenly or suddenly.
You need a spread of food teams. You crave solely bound foods.

You feel the feeling of fullness and take it as a cue to prevent feeding. you will binge on food and not feel a sensation of fullness.

You have no negative feelings regarding feeding. you are feeling guilt or shame regarding feeding.

Physical and emotional hunger is also simply confused, however there are key variations between the 2. listen to however and once your hunger starts similarly as how you are feeling once feeding.

How to stop emotional feeding
Emotional hunger isn't simply squelched by feeding
While filling up may fit within the moment, feeding owing to negative emotions usually leaves folks feeling a lot of upset than before. This cycle usually doesn't finish till someone addresses emotional desires head on.

Find different ways in which to deal with stress
Discovering otherwise to upset negative emotions is usually the primary step toward overcoming emotional feeding. this might mean writing in a very journal, reading a book, or finding some minutes to otherwise relax and decompress from the day.

It takes time to shift your outlook from reaching for food to partaking in different styles of stress relief, thus experiment with a spread of activities to search out what works for you.

Move your body
Some folks realize relief in obtaining regular exercise. A walk or jog round the block or a fix yoga routine could facilitate in notably emotional moments.

In one study, participants were asked to have interaction in eight weeks of yoga. They were then assessed on their attentiveness and perceptive understanding — essentially their understanding of themselves and of things close them.

The results showed that regular yoga is also a helpful preventative live to assist diffuse emotional states like anxiety and depression.

Try meditation
Others are calmed by turning inward to practices like meditation.

There are a spread of studies that support attentiveness meditation as a treatment for binge upset and emotional feeding.

Simple deep respiratory is meditation that you just will do nearly anyplace. Sit in a very quiet house and target your breath — slowly flowing in and out of your nostrils.

You can browse sites like YouTube for free of charge target-hunting meditations. for instance, mythical being Stephenson's "Guided Meditation for Anxiety & Stress" has over four million views and goes through a series of visual image and respiratory exercises for over half-hour.

Start a food diary

Keeping a log of what you eat and after you eat it should assist you determine triggers that cause emotional feeding. you'll be able to jot notes in a very notebook or communicate technology with an app like MyFitnessPal.

While it will be difficult, try and embrace everything you eat — but huge or little — and record the emotions you're feeling in this moment.

Also, if you decide on to hunt medical facilitate regarding your feeding habits, your food diary will be a great tool to share together with your doctor.

Eat a healthy diet
Making sure you get enough nutrients to fuel your body is additionally key. It will be tough to differentiate between true and emotional hunger. If you eat well throughout the day, it should be easier to identify once you're feeding out of tedium or unhappiness or stress.

Still having trouble? attempt reaching for healthy snacks, like contemporary fruit or vegetables, plain popcorn, and different low-fat, low-calorie foods.

Take common things out of your storage room
Consider trashing or donating foods in your cabinets that you just usually reach for in moments of strife. assume high-fat, sweet or calorie-laden things, like chips, chocolate, and frozen dessert. conjointly table journeys to the market once you're feeling upset.

Keeping the foods you crave out of reach once you're feeling emotional could facilitate break the cycle by supplying you with time to assume before noshing.

Pay attention to volume

Resist grabbing an entire bag of chips or different food to snack on. activity out parts and selecting little plates to assist with portion management are conscious feeding habits to figure on developing.

Once you've finished one serving to, offer yourself time before going back for a second. you will even wish to undertake another stress-relieving technique, like deep respiratory, within the meanwhile.

Seek support

Resist isolation in moments of unhappiness or anxiety. Even a fast telephone call to an acquaintance or loved one will do wonders for your mood. There are formal support teams which will facilitate.

Overeaters Anonymous is a corporation that addresses mortal sin from emotional eating, compulsive overeating, and different feeding disorders.

Your doctor could provide you with a referral to a counselor or coach who will assist you determine the emotions at the route of your hunger. realize different teams in your space by looking out on social sites like Meetup.

Banish distractions

You may end up feeding ahead of the tv, computer, or another distraction. attempt change off the tube or putt down your phone succeeding time you discover yourself during this pattern.

By specializing in your food, the bites you're taking, and your level of hunger, you will discover that you're feeding showing emotion. Some even realize it useful to target manduction ten to thirty times before swallowing a bite of food.

CHAPTER 3:

Doing this stuff provides your mind time to catch up to your abdomen.

Work on positive self-talk

F eelings of shame and guilt are related to emotional feeding. It's necessary to figure on the self-talk you expertise once associate episode — or it should cause a cycle of emotional feeding behavior.

Instead of coming back down onerous, attempt learning from your black eye. Use it as a chance to arrange for the long run. And make certain to reward yourself with self-care measures — taking a shower, going for a leisurely walk, then on — after you create strides.

Food could facilitate ease emotions ab initio, however addressing the sentiments behind the hunger is vital within the future. Work to search out other ways to upset stress, like exercise and peer support, and check out active conscious feeding habits.

When to examine your doctor
It's diligence, however attempt gazing your emotional feeding as a chance to urge a lot of connected with yourself and your feelings.

Taking the method day by day can eventually cause an improved understanding of yourself, similarly as toward the event of more healthy feeding habits.

Left unaddressed, emotional feeding could cause binge upset or different eating disorders.

It's necessary to examine your doctor if you are feeling you're feeding patterns are out of your management. Your doctor could refer you to a counselor or dietician to assist address each the mental and physical facet of emotional feeding.

Sometimes the strongest food cravings hit once you're at your weakest purpose showing emotion. you will communicate food for comfort — consciously or unconsciously — once facing a tough drawback, feeling stressed or perhaps feeling bored.

Emotional feeding will sabotage your weight-loss efforts. It usually results in feeding an excessive amount of — particularly too much of high-calorie, sweet and fatty foods. the great news is that if you're susceptible to emotional feeding, you'll be able to take steps to regain management of your feeding habits and find back on course together with your weight-loss goals.

How the food-weight loss cycle works

Emotional feeding is eating as the way to suppress or soothe negative emotions, like stress, anger, fear, boredom, unhappiness and loneliness. Major life events or, a lot of unremarkably, the hassles of existence will trigger negative emotions that cause emotional feeding and disrupt your weight-loss efforts. These triggers would possibly include:

Relationship conflicts

Fatigue

Financial pressures

Health issues

Work or different stressors

Although some folks eat less within the face of robust emotions, if you're in emotional distress you may communicate impulsive or binge feeding, quickly intense whatever's convenient while not enjoyment.

In fact, your emotions will become thus tied to your feeding habits that you just mechanically reach for a treat whenever you're angry or stressed stupidly regarding what you're doing.

Food conjointly is a distraction. If you're troubled regarding a future event or stewing over a conflict, as an example, you will target feeding food rather than addressing the painful state of affairs.

Whatever emotions drive you to eat, the tip result's usually identical. The result is temporary, the emotions come and you probably then bear the extra burden of guilt regarding setting back your weight-loss goal. this will conjointly cause an unhealthy cycle — your emotions trigger you to satiate, you beat yourself up for obtaining off your weight-loss track, you are feeling dangerous and you satiate once more.

Most people assume emotional feeding is because of a scarcity of self-control. However, in my intensive work with feeding disorders and disordered eating, i might say that's seldom the case. If emotional feeding were a straightforward issue of discipline, we tend to might simply realize this discipline while not torturing ourselves over meal plans, paying cash for special diets, and perpetually obsessing regarding who is feeding what and once. And, of course, there would be no feeding disorders.

CHAPTER 4:

How does one go back to on track?

When negative emotions threaten to trigger emotional feeding, you'll be able to take steps to manage cravings. to assist stop emotional feeding, attempt these tips:

Keep a food diary. Write down what you eat, what proportion you eat, after you eat, how you're feeling after you eat and the way hungry you're. Over time, you may see patterns that reveal the association between mood and food.

Tame your stress. If stress contributes to your emotional feeding, attempt a stress management technique, like yoga, meditation or deep respiratory.

Have a hunger reality check. Is your hunger physical or emotional? If you Greek deity simply some hours agone and don't have a rumbling abdomen, you're in all probability not hungry. offer the desire time to pass.

Get support. You're a lot of probably to offer in to emotional feeding if you lack an honest support network. contact family and friends or contemplate connection a support cluster.

Fight tedium. rather than snacking once you're not hungry, distract yourself and substitute a healthier behavior. Take a walk, watch a motion picture, play together with your cat, hear music, read, surf the net or decision an acquaintance.

Take away temptation. Don't keep hard-to-resist comfort foods in your home. And if you are feeling angry or blue, table your trip to the market till you've got your emotions in restraint.

Don't deprive yourself. once making an attempt to reduce, you may limit calories an excessive amount of, eat identical foods repeatedly and banish treats. this might simply serve to extend your food cravings, particularly in response to emotions. Eat satisfying amounts of healthier foods, get pleasure from associate occasional treat and find lots of selection to assist curb cravings.

Snack healthy. If you are feeling the urge to eat between meals, select a healthy snack, like contemporary fruit, vegetables with low-fat dip, kooky or unbuttered popcorn.

Or attempt lower calorie versions of your favorite foods to examine if they satisfy your desire.

Learn from setbacks. If you've got associate episode of emotional feeding, forgive yourself and begin contemporary succeeding day. try and learn from the expertise and create a concept for the way you'll be able to forestall it within the future. target the positive changes you're making in your feeding habits and provides yourself credit for creating changes that'll cause higher health.

What I even have to mention on this subject material isn't original; but, generally a repeating of the knowledge will function a useful reminder. Over and another time, I see the subsequent 5 factors that contribute to emotional feeding.

1. unknowingness

Emotional feeding will be a right away results of not being attentive to what or why you're eating. Therapists decision this unconscious feeding. Unconscious feeding is once you're through with your meal, and you still decide at it, slowly feeding the remaining portion that you just meant to depart behind. It may be putt peanuts or fruity or the other food in your mouth, simply because it's ahead of you.

The solution? try and stay conscious of what and after you are feeding. i do know it will be tedious to focus utterly on your feeding, particularly at first! begin slowly and avoid self-judgment as you are attempting out a replacement manner of being.

2. Food As Your solely Pleasure

I've usually asked folks what they might got to feel if they didn't binge or satiate, and therefore the common answer is, "I would don't have anything to seem forward to." And at the tip of an extended and agitated day, an enormous bowl of frozen dessert will be particularly effective in briefly soothing our exhausted, hard-working selves. Why? in keeping with several sources (e.g. this article), feeding sugars and fats releases opioids in our brains. Opioids are the active ingredients in cocain, heroin, and lots of different narcotics. that the calming, soothing effects you are feeling after you eat frozen dessert and BBQ potato chips are real. And breaking these habits will be like kicking a drug habit.

The solution? realize different ways in which to reward and soothe yourself besides food (and other dangerous behaviors). can these different ways in which be as effective at soothing you as food? fully not! the items you return up with will facilitate somewhat, however so as to actually surrender emotional feeding, you're conjointly aiming to got to apply tolerating tough feelings.

3. Inability to Tolerate tough Feelings

In our culture, we tend to learn from a young age to avoid things that feel dangerous. sadly, the ways in which we've found to distract ourselves from tough feelings aren't forever in our greatest interests. while not the power to tolerate experiencing life's inevitable foul feelings, you're liable to emotional feeding.

The solution? apply lease yourself expertise tough feelings. I know, a lot of easier aforementioned than done! i do know you don't like feeling mad, sad, rejected, and bored. and folks usually solicit from me, "What's the purpose in feeling mad? It doesn't amendment something." Well, it should not amendment the supply of your anger, however it'll forestall you from having to blunt your feelings with behaviors you'd prefer to stop — like feeding.

4. Body Hate

It may sound unreasonable, however it's true: Hating your body is one in all the largest factors in emotional feeding. Negativity, shame, and emotion seldom inspire folks to form long-lived nice changes, particularly once it involves our bodies or our sense of self. many of us tell ME they're going to stop hating their body once they reach their goal weight. I say you've got to prevent hating your body before you'll be able to stop the emotional feeding cycle.

The solution? sadly, this one is multi-layered, complicated, and distinctive for every person. to actually create permanent progress during this space needs over what's potential on behalf of me talk about in a very diary post. Sorry, friends!

5. Physiology

Letting yourself get too hungry or too tired is that the best thanks to leave yourself at risk of emotional feeding. once your body is hungry or tired, it not solely sends robust messages to your brain that signal it to eat, however once we're hungry and tired, we're not on our A game. This leaves us less equipped to defend cravings or urges.

The solution? You guessed it! Get lots of sleep, and eat many little meals throughout the day. (I'm a genius, right?) i do know you're aiming to tell ME that you just don't have time, however if your goal is to prevent emotional feeding, you're aiming to got to create those 2 things a priority. there's no manner around it.

Emotional feeding could be a powerful and effective thanks to realize temporary relief from several of life's challenges. If it didn't work thus well, nobody would get it on. so as to prevent this cycle of emotional feeding, you've got to form a commitment to succeed in deep within yourself to search out an area of grit and strength, and hopefully the higher than reminders will assist you in your journey.

Characteristics of emotional eating

Emotional feeding typically happens once one is trying to satisfy his or her epicurean drive, or the drive to eat palatable food to get pleasure within the absence of an energy deficit however may occur once one is seeking food as a bequest, feeding for social reasons (such as eating at a party), or feeding to evolve (which involves eating as a result of friends or family desires the individual to). once one is partaking in emotional feeding, they're typically seeking out palatable foods (such as sweets) instead of simply food normally. In some cases, emotional feeding can cause one thing referred to as "mindless eating" throughout that the individual is eating while not being conscious of what or what proportion they're consuming; this will occur during each positive and negative settings.

Emotional hunger doesn't originate from the abdomen, like with a rumbling or growling abdomen, however tends to begin once someone is concerned a desire or desires one thing specific to eat. Emotional responses are completely different. Giving in to a desire or feeding owing to stress will cause feelings of regret, shame, or guilt, and these responses tend to be related to emotional hunger. On the opposite hand, satisfying a physical hunger is giving the body the nutrients or calories it must perform and isn't related to negative feelings.

Major theories behind feeding

Current analysis suggests that bound individual factors could increase one's chance of exploitation emotional feeding as a header strategy. The inadequate have an effect on regulation theory posits that people interact in emotional feeding as a result of they believe mortal sin alleviates negative feelings. Escape theory builds upon inadequate have an effect on regulation theory by suggesting that folks not solely satiate to deal with negative emotions, however they realize that mortal sin diverts their attention off from a stimuli that's threatening shallowness to target a pleasant stimuli like food.

Restraint theory suggests that mortal sin as a results of negative emotions happens among people who already restrain their eating. whereas these people usually limit what they eat, once they are round-faced with negative emotions they cope by partaking in emotional feeding. Restraint theory supports the thought that people with different feeding disorders are a lot of probably to have interaction in emotional eating. along these 3 theories counsel that associate individual's aversion to negative emotions, notably negative feelings that arise in response to a threat to the ego or intense awareness, increase the propensity for the individual to utilize emotional feeding as a way of handling this aversion.

The biological stress response may additionally contribute to the event of emotional feeding tendencies. in a very crisis, corticotropin-releasing secretion (CRH) is secreted by the neural structure, suppressing appetency and triggering the discharge of glucocorticoids from the endocrine. These steroid hormones increase appetency and, unlike CRH, stay within the blood for a chronic amount of your time, usually leading to hyperphagia. those that expertise this biologically instigated increase in appetency throughout times of stress are thus fit to have confidence emotional feeding as a header mechanism.

CHAPTER 5:

Contributing factors

Negative effect

Overall, high levels of the negative have an effect on attribute are associated with emotional feeding. Negative affectivity could be a temperament attribute involving negative emotions and poor self-concept. Negative emotions old among negative have an effect on embrace anger, guilt, and nervousness. it's been found that bound negative have an effect on regulation scales expected emotional feeding.

An inability to articulate and determine one's emotions created the individual feel inadequate at regulation negative have an effect on and so a lot of probably to have interaction in emotional feeding as a way for handling those negative emotions. additional scientific studies concerning the link between negative have an effect on and feeding realize that, once experiencing a nerve-wracking event, food consumption is related to reduced feelings of negative have an effect on (i.e. feeling less bad) for those enduring high levels of chronic stress. This relationship between feeding and feeling higher suggests a self-reinforcing alternate pattern between high levels of chronic stress and consumption of extremely palatable foods as a header mechanism. Contrarily, a study conducted. found that negative have an effect on isn't considerably associated with emotional feeding, however the 2 are indirectly associated through emotion-focused header and avoidance-distraction behaviors. whereas the scientific results differed somewhat, they each counsel that negative have an effect on will play a job in emotional feeding however it should be accounted for by different variables.

Childhood development

For some folks, emotional feeding could be a learned behavior. throughout childhood, their oldsters offer them treats to assist them upset a troublesome day or state of affairs, or as a bequest for one thing sensible. Over time, the kid who reaches for a cookie once obtaining a nasty grade on a take a look at could become associate adult who grabs a box of cookies after a rough day at work. In associate example like this, the roots of emotional feeding are deep, which may create breaking the habit very difficult. In some cases, people could eat order to conform; for instance, people is also told "you got to end your plate" and therefore the individual could eat past the purpose during which they feel glad.

Related disorders

Emotional feeding as a way to cope is also a precursor to developing eating disorders like binge eating or bulimia nervosa. the link between emotional feeding and different disorders is basically because of the very fact that emotional eating and these disorders share key characteristics. a lot of specifically, they're each associated with feeling targeted header, maladjustive header ways, and a robust aversion to negative feelings and stimuli. it's necessary to notice that the causative direction has not been definitively established, that means that whereas emotional feeding is taken into account a precursor to those eating disorders, it conjointly is also the consequence of those disorders. The latter hypothesis that emotional feeding happens in response to a different upset is supported by analysis that has shown emotional eating to be a lot of common among people already tormented by bulimia nervosa.

Biological and environmental factors

Stress affects food preferences. various studies — granted, several of them in animals — have shown that physical or emotional distress will increase the intake of food high in fat, sugar, or both, even within the absence of caloric deficits.Once eaten, fat- and sugar-filled foods appear to possess a feedback result that dampens stress connected responses and emotions, as these foods trigger Intropin and opioid releases, that defend against the negative consequences of stress. These foods extremely are "comfort" foods in this they appear to counteract stress, however rat studies demonstrate that intermittent access to and consumption of those extremely palatable foods creates symptoms that jibe opioid withdrawal, suggesting that high-fat and high-sugar foods will become neurologically habit-forming some examples from the yank diet would include: hamburgers, pizza, french-fried potatoes, sausages and savory pasties. the foremost common food preferences are in decreasing order from: sweet energy-dense food, non-sweet energy-dense food then, fruits and vegetables. This might contribute to people's stress-induced looking for those foods.

The stress response could be a highly-individualized reaction and private variations in physiological reactivity may additionally contribute to the event of emotional feeding habits. ladies are a lot of probably than men to resort to feeding as a header mechanism for stress, as are fat people and people with histories of dietary restraint. In one study, ladies were exposed to associate hour-long social agent task or a neutral control. the ladies were exposed to every condition on completely different days. once the tasks, the ladies were invited to a buffet with each healthy and unhealthy snacks. those that had high chronic stress levels and a coffee corticoid reactivity to the acute stress task consumed considerably a lot of calories from cake than ladies with low chronic stress levels once each management and stress conditions. High corticoid levels, together with high hypoglycaemic agent levels, is also accountable for stress-induced feeding, as analysis shows high corticoid reactivity is related to hyperphagia, associate abnormally raised appetency for food, throughout stress.what is more, since glucocorticoids trigger hunger and specifically increase one's appetency for high-fat and high-sugar foods, those whose adrenal glands naturally secrete larger quantities of glucocorticoids in response to a agent are a lot of inclined toward hyperphagia. in addition, those whose bodies need longer to clear the blood of excess glucocorticoids are equally susceptible.

These biological factors will move with environmental components to additional trigger hyperphagia. Frequent intermittent stressors trigger continual, isolated releases of glucocorticoids in intervals too short to permit for a whole come to baseline levels, resulting in sustained and elevated levels of appetency. Therefore, those whose lifestyles or careers entail frequent intermittent stressors over prolonged periods of your time so have larger biological incentive to develop patterns of emotional feeding, that puts them in danger for semipermanent adverse health consequences like weight gain or upset.

Macht (2008) delineated a five-way model to elucidate the reasoning behind nerve-wracking eating: (1) emotional management of food selection, (2) emotional suppression of food intake, (3) impairment of psychological feature feeding controls, (4) feeding to control emotions, and (5) emotion-congruent modulation of feeding. These break down into subgroups of: header, reward improvement, social and conformity motive. Thus, providing a personal with are stronger understanding of private emotional feeding.

Positive have an effect on

Geliebter and Aversa (2003) conducted a study scrutiny people of 3 weight groups: weedy, traditional weight and overweight. each positive and negative emotions were evaluated. once people were experiencing positive emotional states or things, the weedy cluster coverage feeding over the opposite 2 teams. As a proof, the everyday nature of weedy people is to eat less and through times of stress to eat even less. However, once positive emotional states or things arise, people are a lot of probably to indulge themselves with food.

Impact
Emotional feeding could qualify as avoidant header and/or emotion-focused coping. As header ways that fall into these broad classes target temporary reprieve instead of sensible resolution of stressors, they'll initiate a vicious circle of maladjustive behavior bolstered by fugitive relief from stress. In addition, within the presence of high insulin levels characteristic of the recovery section of the stress-response, glucocorticoids trigger the creation of associate catalyst that stores away the nutrients current within the blood once an episode of emotional feeding as visceral fat, or fat set within the abdominal space. thus, those that struggle with emotional feeding are at larger risk for abdominal fatness, that is successively coupled to a larger risk for metabolic and upset.

Treatment

There are various ways in which during which people will scale back emotional distress while not partaking in emotional feeding as a way to cope. the foremost salient selection is to reduce maladjustive header ways and to maximize the adaptive strategies. A study conducted by Corstorphine et al. in 2007 investigated the link between distress tolerance and disordered feeding. These researchers specifically targeted on however completely different header ways impact distress tolerance and disordered feeding. They found that people who have interacted in disordered feeding usually use emotional shunning ways. If a personal is round-faced with robust negative emotions, they will favor to avoid true by distracting themselves through mortal sin. Discouraging emotional shunning is so a very important aspect to emotional feeding treatment. the foremost obvious thanks to limit emotional shunning is to confront {the issue|the difficulty|the drawback} through techniques like problem finding. Corstorphine et al. showed that people who have engaged in drawback finding ways enhance one's ability to tolerate emotional distress.Since emotional distress is correlative to emotional feeding, the power to raised manage one's negative have an effect on ought to permit a personal to deal with a state of affairs while not resorting to mortal sin.

One way to combat emotional feeding is to use attentiveness techniques. For instance, approaching cravings with a nonjudgmental curiosity will facilitate differentiate between hunger and emotionally-driven cravings. a personal could raise his or herself if the desire developed chop-chop, as emotional feeding tends to be triggered ad lib. a personal may additionally take the time to notice his or her bodily sensations, like hunger pangs, and coinciding emotions, like guilt or shame, so as to form aware choices to avoid emotional feeding.

Emotional feeding may be improved by evaluating physical aspects like secretion balance. feminine hormones, above all, will alter cravings and even self-perception of one's body. in addition, emotional feeding will be exacerbated by social pressure to be skinny. the main target on thinness and fasting in our culture will create young women, especially, at risk of falling into food restriction and subsequent emotional feeding behavior.

Emotional upset predisposes people to a lot of serious feeding disorders and physiological complications. Therefore, combatting disordered feeding before such progression takes place has become the main target of the many clinical psychologists.

EMOTIONAL EATING

Break the Cycle, Say STOP Binge Eating! A Proven 21-Day Program Based on Ten Intuitive Principles for a Healthy Relationship with Food. Be Free from the Slavery of Hunger (Part 2)

By
Kelly Francis

© Copyright 2020 - All rights reserved.

The content contained within this book may not be reproduced, duplicated or transmitted without direct written permission from the author or the publisher.

Under no circumstances will any blame or legal responsibility be held against the publisher, or author, for any damages, reparation, or monetary loss due to the information contained within this book. Either directly or indirectly.

Legal Notice:

This book is copyright protected. This book is only for personal use. You cannot amend, distribute, sell, use, quote or paraphrase any part, or the content within this book, without the consent of the author or publisher.

Disclaimer Notice:

Please note the information contained within this document is for educational and entertainment purposes only. All effort has been executed to present accurate, up to date, and reliable, complete information. No warranties of any kind are declared or implied. Readers acknowledge that the author is not engaging in the rendering of legal, financial, medical or professional advice. The content within this book has been derived from various sources. Please consult a licensed professional before attempting any techniques outlined in this book.

By reading this document, the reader agrees that under no circumstances is the author responsible for any losses, direct or indirect, which are incurred as a result of the use of information contained within this document, including, but not limited to, — errors, omissions, or inaccuracies.

INTRODUCTION

Emotional Eating: Break the Cycle, Say STOP Binge Eating! A Proven-Effective 21-Day Program Based On Ten Intuitive Principles For A Healthy Relationship With Food. Find Freedom From Dieting Forever. Emotional eating is described as "the urge to eat in reaction to positive and negative feelings." While the word emotional eating mostly applies to eating as a means of coping with negative emotions, it also includes eating for positive emotions, such as eating food while enjoying an accomplishment or eating to boost an already good mood. Emotions often guide the feeding in these conditions but not in a negative way.

Any people get to terms with difficult situations by having comfort food. Chowing on ice cream or macaroni, and cheese will make it look like it's all right. And maybe there is an explanation why.

As points out, parts of the brain are punished with eating high-fat or high-sugar items. And more than a decade of psychological research shows that any rewarding activity would possibly replicate itself.

Emotional feeding means eating for purposes other than hunger. You can eat for being unhappy, upset, tired or lonely. Or you could be using food as a reward. Nutrition will find you relaxing and divert you from what really does concern you.

Eating comfort food as things get tough — also recognized as emotional eating or eating stress — is not, though, an answer to the challenges of life. It only works briefly. Worse, if it brings on weight gain, it creates longer-term anxiety.

Knowing what causes your emotional eating: Another way to control emotional eating is to find out what the symptoms are. Keep a food diary that not only tracks what you eat and how much but also how you felt at the time.

When you identify a trend, build a turnaround plan. For starters, if you often eat because you believe after a bad day you deserve it, realize that you also deserve to lose weight, feel healthy and be proud of yourself. If you are eating because of tension, learn to turn the discomfort down. Yoga, meditation and regular exercise may help to lower levels of stress.

Reasons of emotional eating: When finding out why you need comfort food you may be able to stop panic eating or emotional eating. Is it calming you down, cheering you up, making up for a bad day or a combination? Recognizing such patterns of thought can promote resistance to giving in. It also helps to understand that emotional eating is not solving the problem that led you to get angry.

The greatest breaks from emotional eating are activities that only require about five minutes switching gears— just long enough to help.

Several suggestions for moving strategies include: walking outside for a five-minute walk, turning on your favorite music and dancing, contacting a close friend to talk. The more ways you will think about entertaining yourself, the better it will become to stop eating tension over time. Instead it will become your new habit of fighting.

If you're an emotional eater, you may not notice the inherent signs of appetite and fullness in your body. You should eat more than you need or wish for. Emotional eating may interfere with making healthy choices regarding food. And it can keep you from getting to and remaining at a healthy weight.

What are symptoms of mental sustenance?

Everybody feeds from time to time, for purposes other than thirst. But if you find that out of hunger or for relaxation you sometimes search for food, you may be consuming for emotional reasons.

Common signs of emotional eating are: if you have more stress in your life, adjust your eating habits.
Feed if you're not thirsty, or are full.
Eating to soothe feelings.
Meat is used as a compliment.
Eating so as not to contend with a stressful situation.

Identify the emotional eating symptoms
One way to find out what emotional eating causes is to keep a diary of food. Factor in when and what you're doing. Write down also what you do and felt before you started eating. To find patterns in your eating habits, you can use this knowledge. For starters, you might find that you purchase an unhealthy snack from the office vending machine any time you start thinking about an assignment at work.

Use a scale of hunger: A scale of hunger will help you learn how to tell the difference between real, actual hunger and hunger in your mind. Psychological appetite is an eating impulse triggered by feelings, such as pain, anxiety, disappointment, or joy.

Value your appetite on a scale of 1 to 10 as you start feeling like you want something to eat, with 1 starving and 10 being so loaded you feel sick. A 5 or 6 rating means that you're comfortable— neither too hungry nor too whole.

Emotional eating is a form of reducing or relaxing negative emotions, such as tension, rage, anxiety, depression, sorrow and loneliness. Major events in life or, more generally, the daily life hassles may cause negative emotions that contribute to emotional eating and hinder the attempts to lose weight.

1—Starving, exhausted, dizzy 2—Very thin, cranky, low-energy, plenty of stomach rumbling 3—Pretty tired, stomach rumbling a little 4—Starting to feel a little better 5—Satisfied, neither hungry nor complete 6—A little full, comfortably full 7—A little awkward 8—Feeling bloated 9—Very cramped, stomach hurts 10—So loaded you feel sick

Use the scale to evaluate your appetite. If you feel like eating but your degree of hunger is a scale 6 or higher, pause and test your emotions.

Unpleasant eating happens when the diet becomes the reaction of an individual to certain unpleasant internal or external signals. The emotional eater may consume comfort foods rather than dealing in their thoughts and the stress they put in in an effort to distract themselves from the pain. This also includes, in most situations, a form of compulsive overeating that results in an overly full stomach sensation. Of reality, consuming this sort of food does not come without negative side effects. Three of the most famous are in the order.

Weight-related health concerns: Depression, high blood pressure, exhaustion and high cholesterol are all health issues that may come from frequent emotional eating outbursts.

Guilt: They're usually filled with guilt and shame for what they've done after the emotional "threat" has passed and the emotional overeater has eaten up. This guilt may contribute to another episode of emotional eating or low self-esteem.

Diarrhea: As nervous eaters often over-eat or eat too fast and suffer stomach pain or diarrhea afterwards, because the sight of food in the stomach acts as a diversion to the feelings they are trying to avoid. It can last a day or two after the actual meal.

We don't forever eat simply to satisfy physical hunger. several folks conjointly communicate food for comfort, stress relief, or to reward ourselves. And after we do, we tend to tend to succeed in for food, sweets, and different comforting however unhealthy foods. you may reach for a pint of frozen dessert once you're feeling down, order a pizza pie if you're bored or lonely, or swing by the drive-through once a nerve-wracking day at work. Emotional feeding is exploitation food to form yourself feel better—to fill emotional desires, instead of your abdomen. sadly, emotional feeding doesn't fix emotional issues. In fact, it always causes you to feel worse. Afterward, not solely will the first emotional issue stay, however you furthermore mght feel guilty for mortal sin.

People who showing emotion eat reach for food many times every week or a lot of to suppress and soothe negative feelings. they will even feel guilt or shame once feeding this manner, resulting in a cycle of excess feeding and associated problems, like weight gain.

The emotional feeding cycle
Occasionally exploitation food as a pick-me-up, a reward, or to celebrate isn't essentially a nasty factor. however once feeding is your primary emotional header mechanism— when your 1st impulse is to open the white goods whenever you're stressed, upset, angry, lonely, exhausted, or bored— you grind to a halt in an unhealthy cycle wherever the important feeling or drawback is rarely addressed .

Emotional hunger can't be crammed with food. feeding could feel sensible within the moment, however the sentiments that triggered the feeding are still there. And you regularly feel worse than you probably did before owing to the uncalled-for calories you've simply consumed. You beat yourself for messing up and not having a lot of resolution.

Compounding the matter, you stop learning healthier ways in which to upset your emotions, you've got a more durable and harder time dominant your weight, and you are feeling more and more overcome over each food and your feelings. however in spite of however overcome you are feeling over food and your feelings, it's potential to form a positive amendment. you'll be able to learn healthier ways in which to upset your emotions, avoid triggers, conquer cravings, and at last place a stop to emotional feeding.

The distinction between emotional hunger and physical hunger

Before you'll be able to become independent from from the cycle of emotional feeding, you initially got to learn the way to differentiate between emotional and physical hunger. this will be trickier than it sounds, particularly if you frequently use food to upset your feelings.

Emotional hunger will be powerful, thus it's simple to mistake it for physical hunger. however there are clues you'll be able to seek for to assist you tell physical and emotional hunger apart.

Emotional hunger comes on suddenly. It hits you in an immediate and feels overwhelming and pressing. Physical hunger, on the opposite hand, comes on a lot of bit by bit.

The urge to eat doesn't feel as dire or demand instant satisfaction (unless you haven't ingested for a awfully long time).

Emotional hunger craves specific comfort foods. once you're physically hungry, nearly something sounds good— including healthy stuff like vegetables. however emotional hunger craves food or sugar-coated snacks that offer an immediate rush. you are feeling such as you would like cheesecake or pizza pie, and zilch else can do.

Emotional hunger usually results in mindless feeding. Before you recognize it, you've ingested an entire bag of chips or an entire pint of frozen dessert while not extremely listening or totally enjoying it. once you're feeding in response to physical hunger, you're usually a lot of awake to what you're doing.

Emotional hunger isn't glad once you're full. you retain wanting a lot of and more, usually feeding till you're uncomfortably stuffed. Physical hunger, on the opposite hand, doesn't got to be stuffed. you are feeling glad once your abdomen is full.

Emotional hunger isn't set within the abdomen. instead of a growling belly or a pang in your abdomen, you are feeling your hunger as a desire you can't get out of your head. You're targeted on specific textures, tastes, and smells.

Emotional hunger usually results in regret, guilt, or shame. after you eat to satisfy physical hunger, you're unlikely to feel guilty or mortified as a result of you're merely giving your body what it desires. If you are feeling guilty once you eat, it's probably as a result of you recognize at bottom that you're not feeding for organic process reasons.
Emotional hunger vs. Physical hunger
Emotional hunger comes on suddenly Physical hunger comes on bit by bit
Emotional hunger looks like it must be glad instantly Physical hunger will wait

Emotional hunger craves specific comfort foods Physical hunger is receptive options—lots of things sound sensible
Emotional hunger isn't glad with a full abdomen. Physical hunger stops once you're full
Emotional feeding triggers feelings of guilt, quality, and shame feeding to satisfy physical hunger doesn't cause you to feel dangerous regarding yourself

Identify your emotional feeding triggers

The first step in putt a stop to emotional feeding is distinctive your personal triggers. What things, places, or feelings cause you to reach for the comfort of food? Most emotional feeding is coupled to unpleasant feelings, however it may be triggered by positive emotions, like appreciated yourself for achieving a goal or celebrating a vacation or blessed event.

CHAPTER 6:

A Simple List of Healthy Living Activities

We have all detected that having healthy habits like feeding well, staying active, and staying on prime of our health screenings is admittedly necessary. But have you ever ever very considered why these items are therefore necessary, and the way all of them work together? The good news is it's not onerous to make healthy, positive activities into your life. notwithstanding however previous you're or how unhealthy your former habits are, you'll be able to consistently introduce tiny changes into what you are doing daily.

Sometimes we are able to check out of management once it involves feeding. we tend to feel compelled to travel on craze diets, or total further onerous at the athletic facility. though it's important to exercise and watch what you eat, it's equally imperative that you just build an honest relationship with food. this could confirm the standard of your life--both at work and reception. Having a healthy relationship with food takes effort however operating towards feeling additional dead with feeding is well worthwhile. Here's what you'll be able to waste order to forestall unhealthy habits from continued.

Be versatile

"Our minds like to suppose in black-and-white terms," says Susan abstract artist, author of fifty ways that to appease Yourself while not Food. "Right versus wrong. Fat versus skinny. excellent versus ruined." If you don a diet, don't let yourself mentally spiral. once this happens, you may end up overthinking, overeating, and even basic cognitive process all types of negative thoughts and judgments regarding yourself. think about being less strict with what you eat. abstract artist advises to even often break your diet--even simply a bit bit--because being versatile will relieve a lot of of the strain you will feel. And, as she notes, "When you see that nothing unhealthy happens, flexibility won't be as discouraging. you may even relish it."

Be attentive.

When does one stuff or eat unhealthy food? will a particular event or feeling trigger your unhealthy feeding habits? typically, for instance, we crave bound foods once we are bored at work, and that we head to the slot machine to resolve the desire. Be aware of your hunger triggers and cues--when you finally notice and concentrate to your unhealthy feeding patterns, you'll be able to effectively dismantle them.

Be relaxed

Keep a relaxed approach once it involves food--not solely will this facilitate with weight maintenance however it conjointly helps you create progress along with your health overall. Relaxed feeding helps you eat till you're nutritionally happy and helps ease emotional eating, therefore think about swiftness down throughout all meals --even lunch at your table. Examine the various textures, tastes, and elements of your food, and higher than all-- enjoy.

What Are Healthy Habits?

A healthy habit is any activity or behavior that may profit your physical, mental, or emotional well-being. At first, these tiny changes may not appear that effective. however once place along dozens of those little habits you'll be able to produce a framework for a healthy life.

It is very important to recollect that healthy habits is created little by little. What may be associate degree unhealthy habit for one person nowadays may be a healthy habit for somebody else.

For example, fake you've got associate degree unhealthy habit of feeding 2 bowls of frozen dessert nightly. Cutting this all the way down to one bowl or perhaps simply 0.5 a bowl is creating progress towards the healthy habit of reducing on unhealthy food. However, for somebody who doesn't eat these foods to start with, feeding a bowl of frozen dessert an evening wouldn't be thought of a healthy habit.

Start wherever you're and build progress towards habits which will be healthy for you.

In this list of healthy habits, you may study feeding higher, exercising, associate degreed having an overall healthy fashion.

While some might not apply to any or all folks, these habits are an excellent start line for anyone who is also trying to raised themselves.

Physical Activity (Fitness)

Getting physical activity edges each your body and your mind. It helps keep your weight up to speed, fights off chronic diseases, reduces stress, improves your mood, and provides you a way of accomplishment.

Getting physical activity doesn't got to involve hours at the athletic facility. Instead, there are many ways that you just will make tiny changes throughout the day to form your life less inactive and acquire your body moving.

You can even involve your friends or family in your physical activity therefore you'll be able to have your time to act with the folks you're keen on while conjointly benefiting your body. There are numerous forms of physical activities that you just may boost your day, it's simply necessary to search out one that you just relish and continue it.

1. Do housekeeping.
2. Take 30-minute early morning walks.
3. Implement the two-minute walking habit for each hour that you just sit.
4. Take the steps rather than the elevator.
5. Walk whenever you'll be able to.
6. Use a treadmill table.

7. Use a height-adjustable table.
8. Aim for 10,000 steps each day. Wear a step-tracking device.
9. Take a dance break.
10. Go hiking additional usually.
11. Do yoga.
12. Go mountain climbing.
13. Go geocaching.
14. exercise throughout TV commercials.
15. Do some Deskercise.

What are the healthiest habits to feature to your routine? Getting physical activity doesn't got to involve hours at the athletic facility. Take a dance break!

Forgiveness (Healthy Lifestyle)
While forgiveness could seem like an antediluvian notion of our rush and quick-to-react society, there are several health edges thereto, even today.

When you are consciously able to let one thing go, even while not associate degree apology, it reduces your anger, stress, and tension.

The physical burden of feeling hurt takes a toll on the body, therefore having the ability to unharness those negative feelings and replace them with quality may be a healthy habit.

Choosing to not forgive somebody will increase your anger and contributes to a sense of loss of management. Holding onto a grudge will increase muscle tension, heart rate, and pressure level, that are all harmful to your health.

Being able to forgive somebody also will improve your sleep. you may not pay time lying in bed in the dead of night ruminating over one thing that happened within the past, or coming up with what quite return you wish to form. If you'll be able to meditate and totally forgive somebody else, you'll be able to focus additional on you and your own well-being. Finally, having the ability to forgive will strengthen your relationship along with your friends and family. Avoiding deep-seeded strains in shut relationships is a crucial a part of feeling connected to those around you and living life harmonical with folks that cross your path. Maintaining healthy relationships may be a key part of living a healthy fashion.

16. Don't move to sleep angry.

17. specialise in understanding yourself rather than blaming others.

18. board this rather than being stuck within the past.

19. get it on for yourself and your own peace of mind.

20. keep in mind the days after you were forgiven.

21. keep in mind folks once they were kids.

22. keep in mind why you're keen on folks.

23. keep in mind that it's higher to be kind rather than right.

24. Observe, don't decide.

25. Take responsibility for your own shortcomings.

26. Acknowledge your growth from the expertise.

Portion Size management (Healthy Eating)

Sometimes, it isn't what you eat, however what quantity of it you're feeding.

For example, avocados are very healthy and have loads to supply in terms of nutrients and healthy fats. However, they're terribly dense in calories, therefore feeding 3 avocados per day wouldn't be a healthy habit.

Eat till you're physically happy, and so stop. If you're thinking that you will still be hungry, wait twenty minutes, drink a glass of water, and rethink if you actually want another serving to.

Also, begin feeding on smaller plates therefore you're feeling as if your plate is full before you sit all the way down to a meal. you may most likely be shocked at the number of food that really accounts for a serving size.

Remember that feeding isn't a pursuit or one thing to try to to after you are bored or wired. confirm you're advertently feeding once it's time to try to to therefore, which you sit down and solely specialise in your food.

Mindlessly feeding ahead of the tv or running to the white goods if you've got had a nasty day are each bad eating habits that cause additional health issues down the road.

27. Avoid feeding once feeling stressed.
28. Use portion-control containers to store your meals.
29. Use portion-control plates once feeding reception.
30. hear your hunger cues.
31. Drink many water and healthy fluids.

32. Keep a food diary or journal.

33. build and drink healthy smoothies.

34. find out how to browse nutrition labels.

35. be from fun-size candy bars and alternative treats.

36. arrange your meals each week.

37. build your own single-serving snack packs.

38. Limit distractions throughout meal times.

39. Take probiotics daily

40. keep on with your grocery list.

41. strive turmeric supplements

42. Take smaller bites and eat slowly.

43. Chew your food a minimum of 5 times before swallowing.

44. Drink before you get thirsty.

healthy living quotes - "An over-indulgence of something, even one thing as pure as water, will intoxicate." — Criss Jami

Preventive Health Care Screening

People tend to travel to the doctor once they become unwell, or once an unacquainted symptom pops up. From there, the doctor works with the patient to treat the matter in hopes that it'll flee. however what if the matter ne'er happened within the 1st place?

For example, if you notice alittle mark on your skin that has ostensibly popped up out of obscurity and you don't understand what it's, this might be a proof of carcinoma that may chop-chop unfold throughout your body. Don't ignore these items and hope they're going to flee. Instead, be proactive and visit a medical specialist each year to induce checkups in order that they will look over your skin for love or money that they'll realize suspicious.

It is necessary to be proactive regarding your health, despite if you're sick or not. Doctors could provide recommendation on preventative measures for diseases that run in your family, or perhaps simply catch a unhealthiness before it becomes too late. Catching health problems early is that the key, therefore confirm that you just are listening to your physical health notwithstanding however you really feel.

43. Annual physical test.
44. Thyroid take a look at (for girls only).
45. Bone mineral density take a look at (women).
46. X ray (women).
47. endoscopy.
48. abstinence plasma aldohexose take a look at.
49. Eye exam.
50. Hearing take a look at.
51. Dental test and improvement.

52. Abdominal aneurism screening (for men only).

53. pressure level screening.

54. sterol screening.

55. Prostate screening (men).

56. carcinoma screening.

57. gonad self-exam (men).

58. Pap test and HPV test (women).

59. Chlamydia take a look at (women).

60. Venus's curse take a look at (women).

61. HIV take a look at and alternative sexually transmitted infection tests.

62. Skin exams.

63. respiratory illness (flu) immunogen.

64. viral hepatitis immunogen.

65. viral hepatitis immunogen.

66. Herpes shingles immunogen.

67. Human papillomavirus (HPV) immunogen.

68. MMR (measles, mumps, rubella).

69. Meningococcal (meningitis).

70. respiratory disorder immunogen.

71. Tetanus, diphtheria, pertussis.

72. chickenpox (chicken pox).

Suggested Timeline for Routine Health Screening

Schedule for men:

Physical exam: each 2 to a few years for men eighteen and over.

Colonoscopy: each 7-10 years for men fifty and over.

Eye exam: One before the age of thirty, as suggested by a doctor when age forty, each one to 2 years when age sixty five.

Hearing test: Once each ten years for men ages 18-50, once each three years for men fifty one and over.

Dental cleaning: double a year for men over eighteen.

Blood pressure screening: each 2 years when the age of eighteen.

Cholesterol screening: each 5 years beginning at age thirty five.

Prostate screening: starting at age fifty.

Skin exam: Yearly, starting at the age of eighteen.

Schedule for women

Physical exam: Annual.

Bone mineral density test: starting at age sixty five.

Mammogram: each one to 2 years beginning at age forty.

Clinical breast exam: each 3 years for ladies Which are 20-40.

Colonoscopy: each 7-10 years for ladies fifty and over.

Fasting plasma aldohexose test: each 3 years starting at age forty five.

Eye exam: One before the age of thirty, as suggested by a doctor when age forty, each one to 2 years when age sixty five.

Dental cleaning: double a year for ladies over eighteen.

Blood pressure screening: each 2 years starting at the age of eighteen.

Cholesterol screening: each 5 years beginning at age thirty five.

Pap test: each 3 years for ladies ages 21-29, each 5 years for ladies 30-65, testing is also discontinued at age sixty five if no previous issues have occurred.

Skin exam: Yearly when the age of eighteen.

Adequate Sleep (Healthy Living)

Sleep plays a awfully necessary role in maintaining general well-being and a healthy fashion. obtaining enough deep sleep in the dead of night will facilitate shield your mental and physical health, your overall quality of life, and your safety.

How you're feeling whereas you're awake is greatly addicted to the standard of sleep you're accessing night. whereas you're sleeping, your body is replenishing itself to support healthy brain perform and optimize your physical health.

Sleep conjointly plays an outsized role within the growth and development of youngsters.

Sleep deficiency will happen each quickly and over time. If you're losing sleep on a daily basis, you will raise your risk for chronic health issues, expertise hassle thinking throughout the day, have delayed reactions, have poor performance at work, expertise learning difficulties, and have issues developing relationships.

If you are doing not provide your body an opportunity to revive itself from expenditure energy all day and prepare itself for the energy you may want the subsequent day, your health will definitely suffer.

73. Avoid alkaloid within the afternoon.
74. Avoid significant meals on the brink of time of day.
75. Keep your pets out of the bed.
76. Be consistent in your sleep schedule.
77. Don't drink too several fluids before bed.
78. Quit smoking.
79. Set your temperature between 60-67 degrees F.
80. Shut off natural philosophy a minimum of associate degree hour before bed.
81. Wear socks.
82. Get non secular.
83. Visualize. suppose happy thoughts.

84. Keep a sleep log.

85. Have a wind-down sleep routine.

86. find out how to induce back to sleep.

87. confirm that the space is dark and quiet.

88. Use an important oil diffuser with the correct volatile oil for sleep.

These healthy habits for adults will assist you start on healthy living and quit smoking.

Give yourself the possibility to sleep higher b quitting smoking and alternative habit-forming substances.

Try one thing New

Everyone gets into a typical routine wherever they are doing constant factor just about a day. However, there are many ways to combine up your schedule a touch therefore you'll be able to strive new things. dynamic your routine can assist you challenge yourself and learn new things.

If you're hesitant initially, you will find yourself shocked at what quantity you relish your new activity or the new folks you meet. making an attempt new things can result in multiplied confidence and a better level of shallowness, whereas conjointly reducing dissatisfaction and loneliness. this may facilitate drive your personal growth, improve your health, and increase longevity.

89. Learn a replacement language.

90. Watch a far off language film (with subtitles, of course).

91. strive feeding at a replacement edifice. Let the waiter perceive your meal.

92. visit somewhere you've ne'er been before.

93. sign on and attend a category associated with your work.

94. strive a replacement sport.

95. Cook a straightforward meal you've ne'er tried before.

96. Take a distinct route to figure, or get there during a new method.

97. Take a road trip.

98. strive a replacement look.

99. hear a replacement (to you) genre of music.

100. browse a book from an author you've ne'er detected of.

101. strive a replacement sort of exercise.

102. Watch a replacement play or musical.

103. Watch a tangle show.

104. Go one week while not web.

105. Go one weekend while not payment.

Strength and adaptability (Fitness)

Your muscles naturally lose strength and reduce in size with age. they're going to doubtless conjointly diminish supple and stiffer. These changes will have an effect on your vary of movement in your joints and cause you to lose tissue snap, which can result in tight muscles.

One of the most reasons that muscles begin to weaken and lose flexibility is inactivity. while not doing strength-building and adaptability exercises, the loss of flexibility could result in permanent harm in your posture and loss of healthy muscle perform. it's so imperative to take care of muscle flexibility as a crucial part of overall fitness.

Having versatile muscles helps to scale back any soreness in your body, and to enhance your posture. Stretching may improve your muscular balance by realigning the tissues in your body, which can cut back the hassle that's required to take care of balance. With robust muscles and adaptability, you may have a diminished risk of injury and a bigger vary of motion.

Finally, active these healthy habits can increase the blood and nutrients that are delivered to the tissues throughout your body. this is often as a result of, after you stretch, you're increasing the temperature of your tissues, that then will increase your circulation and also the transportation of nutrients.

106. Pushups.
107. Crunches.
108. Curl to press.

109. Fly to tris.
110. Lying march.
111. Ball squat.
112. Dips.
113. Tripod row.
114. Shoulder and chest.
115. Arm across chest.
116. striated muscle stretch.
117. striated muscle stretch.
118. skeletal muscle stretch.
119. Single leg hamstring.
120. Standing musculus quadriceps femoris.

healthy fashion quotes - "A work, healthy body—that is that the best fashion statement." —Jess C. Scott

Laugh (Healthy Living)

Some researchers believe that laughter very may be the most effective medication, as a result of it will assist you feel higher and cut back stress. Having a positive angle, being receptive property loose, and having an honest sense of humor also will assist you to develop relationships with people and kind robust bonds.

Studies have truly found that once folks laugh, their brains bear constant changes that they are doing once folks are advertently meditating. This makes folks feel invigorated and prepared to beat issues that they run into throughout the day. The therapeutic worth of laughter remains being studied, but so far, it's solely shown positive results.

121. Learn the therapeutic edges of laughter.
122. plan to happy additional.
123. Watch silly TV shows and flicks.
124. think about finding out a laughter yoga club.
125. be part of a laughter-based exercise program.
126. interact in voluntary, self-initiated laughter.
127. Schedule time to look at funny videos on YouTube.
128. pay longer along with your pets.
129. browse funny books or newspaper comics.
130. Have a favourite comedian.
131. Watch a stand-up comedy show live or on YouTube.
132. hear funny podcasts.
133. join up with previous friends and remember.
134. Visit associate degree common.
135. look into your previous footage.

Family and Friends (Healthy Lifestyle)

We aren't created to measure alone. we tend to are born with our mothers, and quite probably alternative encompassing relations. Throughout numerous stages of life, we rely on people to assist us accomplish things on the method.

In order to try to to most something, you've got to own some kind of cooperation of people. Humans have evolved to collaborate so as to survive. Having each family and friends that you just will consider, turn to, and socialize with can provide you with a way of happiness and permit you to relate to folks that share your values and beliefs.

A very necessary a part of self-care is to form it a priority to develop and maintain human relationships. typically it takes effort throughout our busy lives to stay up-to-date with all of our loved ones, however it's a awfully healthy habit to try to to therefore.

136. build it some extent to eat dinner along as a family.

137. Schedule a weekly family night.

138. Schedule yearly family vacations.

139. Exercise, do chores, and play along.

140. browse time of day stories to young children, and share books with older ones.

141. Keep and still grow your family ikon albums.

142. Get to understand your children's friends.
143. facilitate your children with schoolwork.
144. Go bivouacking along.
145. Bring your children to high school.
146. Leave love or encouraging notes.
147. Work on common goals with (a) friend(s). Be every other's responsibility partner.
148. Host a affair.
149. arrange a reading date along with your friend(s).
150. facilitate your friends with chores.
151. join up with friends for lunch a minimum of once a month.

It's a healthy habit to stay up-to-date with all of our loved ones. build it a priority to develop and maintain human relationships.

Maintaining healthy relationships is one amongst the healthy habits for adults and healthy habits for all times.

Address habit-forming Behaviors

When you accept the word "addiction," you will solely think about alcohol, tobacco, and drug use.

However, there are alternative behaviors that will be healthy sparsely, however that may find yourself turning into addictions. Things like food, caffeine, web usage, and gambling will all become habit-forming for a few folks.

There are safe levels for these forms of behaviors, and that we have to be compelled to acknowledge and address our habits so as to understand once they are in excess. it's necessary to contemplate your temperament once doing this. Studies have shown that there are connections between unthoughtfulness, compulsivity, and addiction.

You have to be able to self-reflect to visualize if you've got any repetitive behaviors that you just do while not a rational motivation.

A full-blown addiction happens after you have associate degree inability to prevent a harmful behavior even if it's negative consequences. If you see a retardant, it's necessary to act to handle the problem.

152. begin by admitting that you just have a retardant.

153. perceive the implications of your habit-forming behavior.

154. Assess however unhealthy your habit-forming behavior is.

155. understand and think about your temperament.

156. Discover what's driving the behavior.

157. perceive your habit loop. establish your triggers. find out how to interrupt unhealthy habits.

158. interact during a new, totally different routine that disrupts your habit-forming behavior.

159. Keep associate degree responsibility journal. (like the liberty Journal)

160. Reward yourself.

161. If you're feeling you wish skilled facilitate, think about seeing a healer.

Quiet Your Mind (Healthy Living)

Taking your time out of the day to quiet your mind and meditate may be a good way to scale back stress. It will assist you connect your body along with your mind and unharness any settled tension from things that are happening in your personal or business life.

This will conjointly provide you with an opportunity to replicate on something happening in your life, and settle for or touch upon issues that are keeping you from being no-hit or achieving your goals. Your mind wants rest throughout the day therefore it is able to strive against ensuing task that comes your method.

162. apply a morning respiration exercise.

163. produce AN "if-then" arrange for times once monkey mind starts to induce the higher of you.

164. apply morning meditation.

165. apply shower meditation.
166. Be an observer of your own thoughts.
167. apply pranayama.
168. apply qigong.
169. begin a journal or write your "morning pages."
170. produce a tea or occasional ritual.
171. apply yoga.
172. Recite mantras or positive affirmations.
173. Build focus.
174. apply aware feeding.
175. Take a digital break often.
176. Take a music break.
177. Decrease distractions.

Gratitude

Reminding yourself what you're grateful for every day can facilitate keep your spirits up and ward off any lingering depression. specialise in the positives in your life instead of the negatives, and keep your strengths in mind as you begin day after day.Making this deliberate purpose of being appreciative for everything you've got in your life is helpful for your happiness and overall well-being. typically we tend to forget the little things that we regard granted a day that we truly wouldn't understand what to try to to while not.

178. Keep a feeling journal.

179. provide a minimum of one compliment a day.

180. Say many thanks

181. Say grace before meals.

182. every morning, think about a minimum of 3 belongings you are grateful for.

183. Smile additional usually.

184. Volunteer for organizations or causes you think in.

185. Write an acquaintance, relative or new acquaintance a many thanks note for being a part of your life.

186. build a feeling collage.

187. Appreciate nature.

188. Listen actively once somebody else is talking.

189. Write and send a many thanks notes.

190. "Look for the helpers." – Fred Rogers

191. Be appreciative after you learn one thing new.

192. Reward effort.

These final list of fine habits for a healthy life embody feeling and spoken communication many thanks as key to a pregnant healthy fashion.

Reminding yourself what you're grateful for every day can facilitate keep your spirits up and ward off any lingering depression.

When you apply healthy habits, you increase your probabilities of living a extended and healthier life. though you begin tiny, you'll be able to considerably cut back your probabilities of developing a chronic unwellness or dying untimely compared with those that apply solely unhealthy habits.

Bad habits could definitely be troublesome to interrupt, however once you're able to get within the routine of active healthy habits, you may not regret your call to form the hassle. whereas your behavioural changes might not occur long, it's necessary to wait and take tiny steps someday at a time.

I hope you enjoyed this in depth list of healthy habits. I hope you're not fazed by the sheer variety of tasks needed to measure a healthy fashion. it's loads, however we tend to don't have to be compelled to be one hundred pc excellent all the time.

If you acknowledge the importance of those healthy habits and do your personal best to incrementally improve you're leagues before those that don't have any plan what healthy living is all regarding.

try these fourteen tips to push durable weight loss and acquire healthier overall—there are numerous edges besides probably nudging the quantity on the scale!

1. concentrate to your parts.

"Most Americans eat 2 to a few times the particular serving size of foods," says Mashru. It doesn't facilitate that restaurants usually serve huge parts, which might train your mind to suppose that's the number of food your body wants. to induce a handle on correct serving sizes, Mashru suggests checking nutrition labels or Googling around to visualize what quantity of any given food counts as some for one person.

2. place your fork down between bites.

It helps you eat additional slowly, that may be a straightforward plan of action to chop back on calories. after you take some time rather than eupnoeic your food, your body will truly register the sensation of fullness, which might take up to twenty minutes to hit your brain. Plus, feeding slowly may even build your food style higher, in keeping with associate degree October 2015 study printed within the journal Proceedings of the National Academy of Sciences of the us of America. Wins all around.

3. drink water 24/7.

Even though your body is mostly a reasonably good machine, it is vulnerable to slip-ups. "Sometimes what you're thinking that may be a hunger pang is caused by thirst," says Zeitlin. That "hunger" will cause you to snack once all of your body needs is a few association. If you're not a lover of the plain stuff, strive these twelve straightforward ways to drink additional water.

4. Carve out time to organize your lunch.

Not solely can creating your own lunch assist you save cash, it'll make sure you understand precisely what you're golf stroke into your body which you're obtaining the correct nutrients. "You're conjointly less doubtless to skip lunch on busy days after you will simply walk to the refrigerator rather than having to travel out and buy," says Mashru. though it feels like skipping those calories may facilitate boost weight loss, depriving your body of normal meals simply causes you to additional doubtless to do it later.

5. Don't do alternative things whereas you're feeding.

It is powerful to specialise in feeding once there's work to try to to and Instagram to ascertain, however chowing down once you're distracted will result in accidentally taking in additional than you wish. Distracted feeding doesn't simply result in additional consumption within the moment, it will even compel you to eat quite necessary afterward within the day, in keeping with a scientific review of twenty four studies within the Feb 2013 edition of The yank Journal of Clinical Nutrition.

CHAPTER 7:

Foods That invariably price but forty Cents Per Serving

Build breakfast a priority. "Eating a breakfast jam-packed with lean supermolecule and fiber can keep you happy, that helps you create higher food decisions throughout the day," to maximise the ability of breakfast, take meals that aren't macromolecule bombs empty substantial to stay you full, like bagels, dry cereal, and muffins. "Try disorganized eggs on whole grain toast, plain Greek dairy product with a cup of your favorite fruit, or associate degree omelette loaded with veggies," says Zeitlin.

Be a sensible nosher.
When you're making an attempt to melt off, snacking will either be your best bud or a ostensibly useful, nonetheless undeniably sneaky saboteur. There's the problem of inadvertently taking in additional than you're thinking that,

that you'll be able to fix during a snap by pre-portioning your snacks in keeping with their serving sizes instead of simply chip away at them every which way. Another snacking drawback will arise if you graze, aka eat senselessly throughout the day, instead of snack advisedly. investigate these snacking for weight loss tips to form positive you're on the correct track.

8. Clock enough hours of sleep nightly.

It is onerous to stay to an honest sleep schedule—especially once there are episodes of state to catch up on—but obtaining enough rest is a simple thanks to encourage weight loss. "Sleep helps keep the appetency hormones hormone and leptin in restraint," "Without AN adequate quantity, those hormones become unbalanced and might result in an multiplied appetency." in keeping with the adults ought to aim for between seven and 9 hours an evening.

Keep on with healthy feeding even on the weekends.

When you're passionate about feeding well Monday through Fri however think about weekends a food scrap, you will not see the burden loss you expect. "If you add it up, feeding poorly and not exertion Fri to Sunday comes dead set twelve days 'off' a month!" says Mashru. "Instead of property the times of the week influence your habits, specialise in making a healthy lifestyle—with the occasional indulgence —that's property all month long."

Consider smaller plates.

If you look into constant quantity of food on a bit plate vs. an outsized one, your eyes may persuade you there's additional appetisingness on the smaller dish. this is often thanks to what's called the Delboeuf illusion, that shows that encompassing one thing during a heap of white area will build it look smaller. though you're not feeding a lot of, curtailing on the number of plate area around your food will trick your brain into thinking it's a much bigger portion than it very is, whereas doing the alternative could tend your hunger by creating you're thinking that you simply Greek deity a touch.

Trim on family vogue feeding.
When you dine with serving dishes jam-packed with further helpings right ahead of you, you'll be able to slip into senselessly filling your plate though you're not still hungry. Instead, whenever doable, limit the food on the table to what you're truly feeding. That's to not say seconds are forbidden—just that you just ought to sign in to visualize if you're still hungry before obtaining up to grab some additional.

Sit facing off from the buffet at restaurants.
Always having additional food in your line of sight could push you to induce into food-coma territory, particularly if you're making an attempt to induce your money's price.

instead of feeding whereas gazing at what you may treat yourself to next, flip your back to the opposite food and specialise in very enjoying what's on your plate. If you wish additional food once you're done, the buffet can still be there!

Pile your plate high with vegetables.
One of the most effective ways that to induce into the healthy-eating habit is by adding things to your diet rather than removing them. Refusing to eat any of your favorite treats will backfire during a binge, whereas slowly increasing your vegetable intake will solely bring smart results. "Not solely are vegetables crammed with necessary nutrients that keep your body healthy and energized, they contain fiber, that helps you're feeling surfeited," says Mashru. To avoid vegetable burnout, she suggests beginning small: add a cup of them to a minimum of one meal each day for per week, then begin incorporating them into additional meals as you get accustomed them.

Keep a food journal.

If you're doing all of the higher than however still not seeing any noticeable weight loss, dropping pounds will want a mysterious equation you only can't crack. in this case, Zeitlin suggests keeping a food journal therefore you've got a close nonetheless overarching read of your habits. "It will assist you realize the areas specific to you and your fashion that would use some tiny tweaking," she says. Do your best to trace your food and potable intake for per week, then recall to visualize if you're inadvertently taking during a few further calories you may cut get in order to induce the results you're when. Above all, keep in mind that losing weight healthily usually involves some trial and error—but the purpose is that on the method you find out how to be smart to your body, that is admittedly what matters.

The Next Healthy Habits you must Build

1. Drink a glass of water very first thing within the morning. This health tip is easy, however conjointly quite necessary. Here are many reasons why this could be a part of your healthy consumption habits:

While sleeping, your body gets dehydrated. What it craves, and can be happy to receive as shortly as attainable, could be a whole glass of water. In giving that to your body, you'll feel instantly invigorated and can conjointly jump begin your metabolism. It seems, you don't essentially have to be compelled to eat breakfast super early, however you doneed to place this supernatural liquid in your system in real time.

To make it even easier, place the glass next to your bed as a reminder. within the morning, fill it with water, add a lemon, and provides yourself concerning five minutes to totally fancy the method of provision your body and brain. build it a meditation! Why not?

Some a lot of advantages of this tiny trick are that it clears your mind and causes you to alert and totally awake. With that, you'll be able to simply begin the day, have a productive morning, and be a lot of centered than usual for the remainder of the day.

Water conjointly helps flush toxins out of the body, strengthens the system, and plays a large role in managing your weight.

Try doing this very first thing within the morning tomorrow and knowledge all of those positive effects for yourself!

CHAPTER 8:

Tiny Healthy habits

2. Leave technology behind within the evening

Most people have sleeping issues. However, it's crucial to induce your eight roughly hours of sleep nightly so as to possess energy and a transparent mind succeeding day. If you don't, your body and brain can suffer in many alternative ways that.

Some of the factors symptom your sleep are attending to bed together with your phone, browsing the net on your laptop computer, observance a pic to induce yourself to sleep, or checking social media and obtaining flooded. For this, victimisation technology before time of day has become a difficulty — it keeps your brain activated; no marvel you have got issues falling asleep.

There's a straightforward answer, and you must add it to your arsenal of daily healthy habits: undo an hour before bed.

Do it for simply ten minutes these days, or advice yourself you won't be taking your phone or laptop computer to bed any longer. Then, build this era of your time longer once you're feeling comfy with it.

It's most higher to travel to bed peacefully and be positive concerning tomorrow, instead of be unbroken awake considering the posts you simply browse on your friend's timeline, the unhealthy news you were bombarded with, or an argument you had on social media.

3. Forming healthy consumption habits with very little changes

You can modification your whole design over time by setting out to for a few little healthy consumption habits these days. for example, you'll be able to begin intense proteins and veggies with every meal. Then, your want for unhealthy foods can eventually get away, and you'll still feel full and happy once an enormous meal.

Soon after, you'll be able to add supplements like polyunsaturated fatty acid fatty acids to your daily diet. It's a little, 2-second act (taking the pills), however are some things which will boost your health in varied other ways. The krill/fish supplement is verified to regulate many sorts of diseases. As a bonus, it fights depression and anxiety, is sweet for your eyes and heart, and reduces inflammation.

4. Journal your thoughts

Journaling is on this list of health tips for many reasons.

First of all, it's another likelihood to remain far from technology and boost your psychological state by removal your mind and swing it all on paper. However, the good thing about this healthy habit goes abundant more.

By sharing your thoughts on paper, you're learning a way to open up. In real world, that creates your relationships better over time and you become a far better person.

It's nice for staying intended to achieve your goals. By writing concerning your goals, you visualize that it's already happening and your brain works to bring you the required circumstances in life to induce you nearer to it vision.

Journaling is additionally a medical care. you'll be able to write your fears and doubts, and feel higher after. It brings clarity and attentiveness to any or all problems you address.

5. Have stretch breaks

This one is for mental and physical health.

The truth is, we tend to work an excessive amount of and don't take breaks — whichs finishes up truly devastation our productivity.

Instead, our brain must be engaged in restful activities the maximum amount as once each hour. that may be as very little as five minutes of stretching, respiratory deeply, enjoying a cup of tea, and simply filling your mind with positive thoughts.

It's conjointly instructed to try and do correct stretching once you get up, and before you visit sleep. within the morning, stretching helps to induce the body get in active mode. within the evening, on the opposite hand, it helps your brain get into sleep mode and is a lot of of a soothing activity, instead of one transfer energy to any or all elements of your body.

6. begin walking

Sounds easy, right? Yet, we tend to avoid it the maximum amount as attainable. Well, currently can be the proper time in your life to feature walking to your daily healthy habits.

It's helpful for your physical well-being as by doing it daily, you're staying active. Also, it's nice for removal your mind, respiratory some contemporary air, obtaining some fat-soluble vitamin (if done throughout the day), and boosting your mood naturally and feeling a lot of alive!

Walking is additionally connected to stronger bones and lower vital sign. If you're not the kind of one that likes exercise, this can be the simplest variety of moving your body and still obtaining the advantages like losing body fat, doing basic cardio, and rising your heart health.

If you're questioning a way to embody it in your daily schedule, you'll be able to do this:

If you get up earlier, it may be an incredible begin of the day. You'll be intended to feature another healthy habits to your morning routine later on.

Even your lunch break may be your formula for achievement at work... If you are doing the proper activities throughout it. this can be as a result of it's necessary to fully shut your brain off and stop considering the items happening at the office; for this, you must do one thing completely different, and ideally outside. If you get out and simply walk, although it's for ten minutes, you'll see that the strain goes away, creating area for relaxation, attentiveness, and even creativeness. Once you're back to figure, you'll realize it easier to focus and can get a lot of done.

7. Prepare your food

If you wish to require care of your well-being, you must accept sensible foods. Don't simply ditch food, even be conscious of what you're fitting your body: live it, have mounted times for meals, and prepare it yourself.

This will all happen over time, of course. Such healthy consumption habits, however, can impact the remainder of your life. Researchers have found that home change of state results in healthier living.

But wait! There's a lot of...
You're building discipline by locution no to consumption on the go. you furthermore mght build have the benefit of shopping for groceries yourself and so obtaining artistic within the room. This method makes the meal one thing to appreciate— you build a brand new talent, track your intake, and therefore the food satisfies you far more currently that you've worked it.

You don't have to be compelled to get something that comes in a very package. Finally begin victimisation your room. You'll shortly begin researching a lot of health tips yourself, what ingredients to incorporate, a way to mix foods, etc.

Such a conscious preparation, and therefore the delicious meal that follows, are nice ways that to stay your relationship together with your loved ones, family, or roommates sturdy (they can love you!). Meals are an opportunity to bond, and consumption is far a lot of pleasant once it becomes a group action. No want for fancy restaurants — you're saving cash by change of state your food, too.

These healthy habits are going to be enough to alter your life in many ways. Begin these days. By shopping for polyunsaturated fatty acid, by swing a glass beside your bed, by journaling many thoughts, or by obtaining outside and walking round the neighborhood for ten minutes. . . you'll feel it.

To live healthy is simple. simply build these a part of your daily routine.

What works for one person might not work for succeeding.

When creating changes, some individuals (like me) choose to go all-in and alter everything at identical time.

But others like the longer, slower approach... creating little changes, one at a time.

Neither approach is healthier than the opposite, it's simply that individuals have completely different personalities and wish to approach mode changes otherwise.

It explains a way to adopt a healthy, real food based mostly diet in twelve easy, simply manageable steps.

You can do one step per week, one each fortnight, or one per month... whichever suits you. Waiting till you get accustomed one modification before creating succeeding could be a sensible plan.

Whatever you are doing, you must begin seeing results at once, as a result of every step will have a strong impact.

When you're through with this, you must have lost a major quantity of weight and improved your health, each physical and mental, in each method conceivable.

Remember... habit puts resolve on autopilot. Changes in mode and behavior may be robust within the starting, however become easy after you flip them into a habit.

By mastering one little habit at a time, you'll set yourself up for long success.

Here are steps to nutrition.

1. Eat a lot of macromolecule to spice up Your Metabolism and cut back Your appetency, creating Future Changes Easier

Before we tend to cipher, we add.

This initiative can modification your metabolism in a very method that creates resultant changes easier.

First of all, macromolecule truly boosts your rate... that is, what percentage calories you burn at rest.

The studies show that top macromolecule diets boost metabolism by eighty to a hundred calories per day, compared to low macromolecule diets.

Second of all, macromolecule will cut back your appetency, creating you mechanically eat less of alternative calorie

In one study, consumption macromolecule at 30% of calories caused an automatic reduction in calorie intake of 449 calories per day. The individuals lost four.9 weight unit (11 lbs) in twelve weeks, while not designedly limiting something,

Of course... adequate macromolecule conjointly has several alternative advantages, together with enlarged muscle mass, stronger bones, lower vital sign, to call many.

Good macromolecule sources embody meat, poultry, fish, seafood, eggs and full-fat dairy farm product (if you'll be able to tolerate them). Some individuals like beans and legumes, that are fully fine if properly ready.

I recommend consumption concerning one.5-2.5 grams of macromolecule per metric weight unit of bodyweight, or 0.7 -1.1 grams per pound.

You don't really want to weigh or live this, however it's going to be an honest plan to trace your foods within the setting out to ensure you're obtaining enough.

Eating a lot of macromolecule is that the best, simplest and most delicious thanks to provide your metabolism a nudge towards a lower weight, reduced appetency and higher health. it'll conjointly build the remainder of the changes easier.

Adding a lot of protein to your diet can boost your metabolism and cut back your appetency, giving your metabolism a nudge and creating resultant changes abundant easier.

2. begin consumption a Healthy Breakfast, ideally With Eggs

The second step involves dynamical one in every of your daily meals... breakfast.

Most people are consumption cereal or one thing similar for breakfast, however that actualy is that the worst issue you'll be able to erode the beginning of the day.

Most breakfast cereals are loaded with refined carbs and sugar (even the healthy trying ones).

Eating these items for breakfast can spike your glucose, resulting in a crash many hours later... followed by cravings for one more high-carb meal (9).

Instead, eat eggs for breakfast.

Eggs are just about the proper food... they're high in macromolecule, healthy fats and contain a large amount of nutrients.

There are many studies showing that if you replace a grain-based breakfast (bagels) with eggs, it will assist you lose fat.

Eggs are best served with vegetables or a fruit... however you'll be able to have quality bacon with them if you wish.

If you can't eat eggs for a few reason, any high-protein, nutrient dense food can answer.

There extremely is not any valid excuse to not eat a healthy breakfast. Once you get this into a routine, getting ready an egg-based breakfast doesn't take over 5-10 minutes, at most. simply set your alarm a small amount earlier.

That being aforesaid, there's no have to be compelled to eat breakfast within the morning if you don't want it, simply ensure that your 1st meal of the day could be a healthy one. Eating a healthy, nutrient-dense breakfast with macromolecule and healthy fats is that the best thanks to begin the day.

3. Replace shitty Fats and Oils With sensible Fats and Oils

Simply substitution unhealthy fats and oils with healthier ones will have a significant impact on your health down the road.

Most people are consumption tons of seriously unhealthy fats... together with trans fats and refined vegetable oils.

Although trans fat consumption has gone down within the past few years and decades, it's still method too high.

To avoid trans fats, ensure you browse the label on something you eat. If it says "hydrogenated" or "partially hydrogenated" anyplace on the label, avoid it.

Refined vegetable oils are problematic. they need a distinct composition than alternative a lot of natural fats, being by artificial means high in omega-6 fatty acid fatty acids. This includes vegetable oil, vegetable oil, vegetable oil and several other others.

Without moving into the main points (you will examine them here), intense vegetable oils is also resulting in enlarged inflammation and aerophilous injury within the body, probably raising your risk of cardiopathy and cancer.

Instead of these nasty fats and oils, opt for fats that are largely saturated and/or monounsaturated. Grass-fed butter, oil, olive oil, avocado oil et al. Whole fruity are a superb supply of fat furthermore.

The comparatively easy act of substitution trans fats and high omega-6 fatty acid vegetable oils with healthy, ancient fats ought to cause some pretty spectacular health advantages and build your body perform higher.

4. take away Sugar-Sweetened Beverages and Fruit Juices From Your Diet

Sugar is unhealthy news... however sugar consumed in a very liquid kind is even worse.

Studies show that the brain willn't "register" liquid sugar calories within the same method because it does calories from alternative foods.

So you may drink many hundred calories of soda in someday (not uncommon), however your brain doesn't take them under consideration once it's attempting to regulate your energy

If you were to feature an entire food to your diet, you'd mechanically eat less of alternative foods instead. In alternative words, your brain would "compensate" for those additional calories.

That doesn't happen with liquid sugar calories. Your brain doesn't complete them, therefore you finish up taking in additional than you would like.

One study shows that intense one serving of sugar-sweetened beverages per day is coupled to a 60% enlarged risk of avoirdupois in kids.

Many alternative studies support this... sugar-sweetened beverages is also the foremost finished facet of the trendy diet.

Keep in mind that potable is simply as unhealthy. It contains identical quantity of sugar as a syrupy drinkable.

Sugar is also the one worst ingredient within the trendy diet, however intense it in a very liquid kind is even worse.

5. begin exercise... realize one thing that you just fancy and may keep on with

Exercise is one in every of the foremost necessary belongings you will do for each physical and psychological state, furthermore as sickness interference.

On its own, it's unlikely to guide to important weight loss.

However... it will facilitate improve your body composition. you'll not be losing weight, however you'll be losing some fat and gaining a small amount of muscle instead.

Exercise results in such a lot of advantages that it's on the far side the scope of this text to list all of them... however let's simply say that exercise is extremely protecting against just about any chronic, Western sickness.

It is conjointly implausibly helpful for mood, well-being and avoiding depression, that could be a quite common downside these days.

When it involves exercise, what you are doing specifically isn't that necessary. what's necessary is finding one thing that you just fancy doing and may keep on with within the long-standing time.

Although a mixture of vessel exercise and a few sort of resistance coaching is also the most effective, one thing as easy as walking conjointly has implausibly powerful health advantages.

If you've already done steps 1-4, the perform of your hormones ought to have improved and your energy levels enlarged, therefore beginning An exercise program might not be that arduous.

Work your high to performing some form of exercise a minimum of three times per week.

Exercise is simply as necessary as nutrition once it involves optimum health. It will improve each physical and psychological state, whereas being extremely protecting against latest, chronic diseases.

6. Replace Sugar, Refined Carbs and trendy Wheat With alternative Healthier Foods

Time to induce eliminate all the "bad" carbs.

Sugar and refined carbs are a number of the unhealthiest aspects of the trendy diet.

They're low in nutrients and fiber and contribute to gluttony, that brings with it a excessiveness of metabolic issues and diseases.

Wheat is in a very league of its own. trendy dwarf wheat, introduced around 1960, is low in nutrients compared to older types of wheat and is far worse for celiac patients and protein sensitive people than older types of wheat.

Instead of the "bad" carbs, opt for healthier carb sources instead. Vegetables, fruits, potatoes, sweet potatoes, healthier grains like rice, oats and quinoa, even legumes if you'll be able to tolerate them.

Whatever you are doing, simply get eliminate the sugar and processed carbs from your diet. Eat real food instead.

Sugar and refined carbs are a number of the foremost damaging aspects of the trendy diet. It's time to induce eliminate them and eat healthier carbs instead.

7. begin consumption Meat or Fish and lots of Vegetables for Dinner

Now it's time to remodel another one in every of your daily meals... dinner.

Replace no matter it's that you're consumption with a meal supported either meat or fish, at the side of lots of wholesome vegetables.

I realize that dinner is that the best meal to suit in lots of veggies.

If you fancy starches (like potatoes or rice) with dinner, then be at liberty to eat those too.

Definitely attempt to eat fatty fish a minimum of 1-2 times per week for all the super healthy Omega-3s. If you can't or won't eat fatty fish, then supplement with animal oil.

Start consumption a healthy dinner supported meat or fish, with lots of vegetables. attempt to eat fatty fish a minimum of 1-2 times per week.

8. Match Carb Intake to Your Metabolic Health and Activity Levels

Carbs are a extremely polemic nutrient.

Some assume the most important a part of our diet ought to be coming back from carbs, whereas others assume they're downright unhealthful.

As with most things, the reality is somewhere in between and depends greatly on the individual.

The optimum carb intake for anyone individual depends on several factors... together with metabolic health, activity levels, food culture and private preference.

Whereas somebody who is lean, healthy and lifts weights five times every week might perform well consumption tons of carbs, somebody who is overweight and doesn't exercise abundant can most likely do higher with a low-carb diet.

Although there's no scientific paper that explains specifically a way to match sugar intake to individual desires, I've in person found these pointers to be effective:

100–150 grams: those that are lean, healthy and physically active (some individuals might have even over this).

50–100 grams: those that are overweight and/or don't exercise abundant.

20–50 grams: those that have tons of weight to lose, or have metabolic issues like sort a pair of polygenic disorder. If weight loss is your goal, you'll be able to slowly add back in healthier carb sources after you reach your ideal weight.

Some individuals perform best consumption lots of carbohydrates. For others, low-carb diets have life saving advantages. It's necessary to match sugar intake to your individual desires and preferences.

9. lookout of Your mode... accenting Adequate Sleep and Reduced Stress Levels

Often unnoticed, sleep and stress levels will have a significant impact on your health.

Studies show that not obtaining enough sleep is powerfully coupled to several serious diseases, together with avoirdupois (34, 35).

Short sleep length may very well be one in every of the strongest risk issue for weight gain. it's coupled to a 55% enlarged risk of avoirdupois in adults and 89% in kids (36Trusted Source).

There are many ways to boost sleep... like sleeping in a very fully dark area, avoiding caffein within the afternoon and evening, furthermore as maintaining an identical sleep schedule.

Another major mode issue is chronic stress.

Excess stress raises your levels of the secretion adrenal cortical steroid, which might cause you to gain tons of fat within the abdomen and lift your risk of all kinds of health issues down the road (37, 38Trusted Source).

Unfortunately, stress may be arduous to wear down. several people are flooded with numerous duties and worries.

Meditation will facilitate with this, however if you're severely stressed all the time and can't realize some way to alter it on your own, then it's going to be an honest plan to hunt skilled facilitate.

Lifestyle factors like obtaining adequate sleep and avoiding chronic stress are implausibly necessary for optimum health, however usually unnoticed.

10. begin consumption Healthy Lunches and Snacks... currently every of Your Daily Meals ought to Be Healthy and wholesome

Now that you've already taken care of breakfast and dinner, it's time to maneuver on to lunches and snacks.

These meals tend to be the foremost problematic for tons of individuals, as a result of they're usually eaten far from home.

A good thanks to perpetually make sure you will eat one thing healthy for lunch is to cook an excessive quantity at dinner, therefore you'll be able to eat leftovers for lunch succeeding day.

But today, as a result of the planet is a lot of health acutely aware than ever before, "fast food" places that serve healthy food have started showing everywhere the place.

It might be an honest plan to jot down down an inventory of places that serve healthier foods, therefore you mostly have some choices accessible if you discover yourself hungry far from home.

Snacks are pretty straightforward... a chunk of fruit and one or two of fruity works well. many arduous cooked eggs, a bag of baby carrots... all of those are simply transportable.

Chances are that you just won't even want snacks at now, since avoiding sugar and processed carbs tends to cut back hunger and cause stable energy levels.

It's time to start out consumption healthy lunches and snacks each day. currently every of your meals ought to be healthy and wholesome. It will facilitate to arrange ahead and have an inventory of "fast food" places that serve healthy foods.

11. Cut Out All Processed Foods and begin specializing in Quality

Now it's time to travel fully real food based mostly.

You should already be 90% there, however if you've been hanging on to something that you just assume is also doing you hurt, now's the time to induce eliminate it.

Clear out your larder... throw away all soda, bread, cereals, flour, sugars, pastries and processed foods. Start specializing in quality ingredients... seek for quality sources of animal foods, opt for grass-fed if you'll be able to.

Eat quality manufacture and check out to avoid any food with artificial ingredients.

Remember... real food doesn't want an ingredients list, as a result of real food is that the ingredient.

It's time to clear your house of all unhealthy, artificial stuff. begin specializing in quality, unprocessed foods at each meal. seek for the healthiest sources of plants and animals.

12. attempt to a lifespan of Improvement

Turn health and nutrition into a hobby.

Subscribe to some blogs and check out to browse many health connected books annually.

Stay health acutely aware for the remainder of your life and you'll live longer, look higher and avoid most of the chronic diseases that individuals suffer from in maturity.

There's a fine line between thinking rigorously concerning what we tend to place into our bodies and obsessing over it or limiting it hazardously.

Whether our explicit issue is emotional consumption, binge consumption, disordered consumption or we tend to simply can't appear to induce a handle on the entire nutrition issue, we will all stand to find out many things from the individuals for whom healthy consumption simply comes simply. Here are many of the items they are doing otherwise.

1. individuals with a healthy relationship to food eat heedfully.

Our body has some pretty important intrinsic cues to inform once to eat -- and when to prevent consumption. however we're not perpetually listening. The follow of participating all of our senses to guide our consumption-related choices is named conscious eating for conscious consumption. conscious consumption will facilitate "acknowledge our response to food while not moving into judgement".

2. They swear by everything -- affirmative, everything -- sparsely.
The Essential Guide To Taking Care Of Your Mind And Body
Morality hooked up to food might stem from the very fact that some religions do have prohibitions once it involves food, he says. Take, as an example, however "some foods are delineated as sinfully delicious," he says.
"It isn't food that's sensible or unhealthy, it's our expertise," says dramatist. "And that's not judgement, it's categorizing." Recognizing foods and consumption things that you just realize pleasant will facilitate inform your future decisions, she says. individuals with a healthy relationship to food tell themselves, "'Eating could be a likelihood on behalf of me to nourish and nurture my

being,'" she says, "as critical, 'I have to be compelled to eat this fashion or those foods.'"

3. however they recognize the temporal order should be right.

However, if you are doing decide you're within the mood for fries or dish or chocolate, says Abramson, fancy your choose at a time once you're not hungry for a full meal, therefore you don't make it. "If you're starving and so you're confronted with a favourite food, you'll consume tons a lot of of it," he says. "Let's say, if you have got it for sweet, you already had your meal, your tummy is full, you'll be able to extremely appreciate the sensations that chocolate provides."

4. They eat once they're physically hungry.

"Emotional consumption is often to assuage unpleasant arousal," says Abramson. sadly, stress and anxiety usually cause us to crave higher-calorie, fattier foods and "most people don't want further caloric intake," he says.

When we use food to do to assuage an feeling, he adds, we tend to mask what that feeling is attempting to show us, and instead replace it with regret or guilt for consumption no matter we tend to grabbed.

5. and that they stop consumption once they're well full.

Hunger and repletion each start up little and grow larger and louder, says dramatist. "Some people don't hear hunger or fullness till it's screaming in our ears," she says. however being more tuned-in whereas consumption will facilitate us "hear" higher furthermore. "Mindfulness is locution, 'I'm attending to listen tougher to my hunger and listen to it once it's not yelling at me, and I'm attending to listen tougher to my fullness therefore it's not yelling at me [either].'" each hunger and fullness modification once each bite, therefore listening in will assist you realize the extent of fullness wherever it's comfy for you to prevent consumption, she says.

6. They eat breakfast.

Regular breakfast eaters have a lot of energy, higher reminiscences and lower sterol. They conjointly feel healthier overall and are usually throw than their peers that don't eat a morning meal. "Starting your day with a healthy, balanced breakfast with proteins, fats and carbs and not high in sugar is that the key to healthy consumption," says Marjorie Nolan plant scientist, MS, RD, CDN, a advocator for the Academy of Nutrition & bioscience and therefore the author of Overcoming Binge consumption For Dummies.

7. They don't keep problematic foods within the house.

Once you recognize your specific patterns of emotional consumption, says Abramson, you'll be able to take little steps to send them. One strategy he recommends is not any longer keeping a very tempting food within the house, therefore you'd have to be compelled to leave home once dinner to induce a style. If, as an example, you actually love frozen dessert, "rather than having it sitting within the deep freezer occupation your name," he says, a handful of times every week, withdraw for frozen dessert.

8. They don't sit down with the entire bag.

Hitting up your native frozen dessert search conjointly has the good thing about providing your treat in a very single serving size. "If you have got a cup or a cone you recognize once you're finished, as critical sitting there having one containerful once another" straight out of the carton, says Abramson. shopping for single-serving packages of your favorite chips or cookies may also facilitate, he says, as will merely serving yourself in a very cup or bowl instead of sitting down with an entire family-size bag of chips.

9. They recognize the distinction between a snack and a treat.

Letting yourself get too hungry could be a instruction for gluttony -- particularly those foods you most wish to stay to smaller parts. Snacking could be a good thanks to ensure you're not ravenous return suppertime. however snack alternative is crucial to each keeping you full and keeping your healthy consumption plans not off course, says Abramson. "A treat is only for enjoyment, whereas a snack are some things you eat between meals to ward off hunger," he says. "Nuts or fruit or cheese may be an honest snack," he says, however chocolate? A treat.

10. they offer themselves permission to fancy consumption.

These tips aren't plausible if we tend to don't build time to price our relationships with food. "So persistently we tend to forget to require the time to eat, and consumption will take time," says dramatist.

She suggests trying ahead at your day and ensuring you have got enough time sculptured bent eat, instead of going to scarf one thing down within the 3 minutes you have got between afternoon conferences. "We build it 3 minutes, which might feed you, however will it nourish you?" she asks. And it's not concerning feeling guilty for missing one thing else by creating time to eat, she says. It's concerning really basic cognitive process we tend to are "worth sitting down and consumption food."

11. They don't "make up" for a meal.

When we realize ourselves feeling guilty a few food alternative, "there's this instinct to create up for it by either overdoing it at the athletic facility or being terribly restrictive at succeeding meal," says plant scientist. Instead, she suggests thinking of this method as a a lot of refined "balancing out". individuals with healthy relationships to food can have a lighter meal later within the day if they attempt to indulge at brunch, as an example, however they won't limit that later meal most in order that they find yourself binging later as a result of they've created themselves too hungry. "You will balance out slowly over the course of every week, however you can't form up among identical day," says plant scientist.

12. They don't eat to check the dimensions shift.

Ideally, we'd all eat what makes us feel sensible, says Cohn. We'd choose the foods that gave us energy to fuel our daily activity, and we'd avoid foods that, say, gave us stomach upset, despite however sensible they tasted, instead of restructuring our consumption plans to create the quantity on the dimensions modification.

13. They're not frightened of feeling hungry.

One of the foremost restrictive patterns of thought that plant scientist sees among purchasers could be a concern of consumption an excessive amount of and consequently gaining weight. "People who have a way of what their body desires and eat heedfully and intuitively once they will, they're not as frightened of their hunger," she says. "What's there to be afraid of? If you get hungry, you simply eat something!"

Some things can't be controlled (your age, case history of diseases, gender). however others will. and people things aren't a large surprise — you already understand to not smoke, drink an excessive amount of, or eat crappily.

It's fascinating, though, however all of the main diseases are caused by constant things: smoking, diet, exercise, alcohol and stress.

Below I'll list the highest habits you'll amendment, and a straightforward methodology for dynamical them.

The Habits of Healthy Living

1. Stop smoking. this can be far and away the foremost vital habit, because it affects virtually each single one amongst the leading causes of death. It's conjointly the toughest of those habits to vary. It's not the least bit not possible — I quit six years past next month (read my tips).

2. change state (if you're overweight). this can be not precisely a habit — the most effective habit to create to change state is to eat less. Or eat a lot of of things that don't have tons of calories, like fruits and veggies. Being overweight is simply below smoking the worst risk issue for several diseases.

3. Exercise. You don't would like ME to inform you to exercise, however hear this: lack of exercise may be a major risk issue for cardiovascular disease, stroke, colon & body part cancers, diabetes, carcinoma, high pressure and high steroid alcohol. If you don't exercise, you're simply asking to urge a serious unwellness. It's virtually a magic pill: do a touch of exercise a day, and you get healthy. You don't would like a lot of — begin with five minutes on a daily basis within the morning.

4. Drink solely carefully. serious drinking is one amongst the worst risk factors for several diseases. That's quite a pair of drinks of alcohol on a daily basis for men, and quite one drink for ladies. A glass of vino may be a sensible factor, however too several and you're greatly increasing your risk of unwellness.

5. Cut out red & processed meats. consumption red meats, and processed meats like sausages, bacon, canned meats so on, may be a risk issue for colon/rectal cancer, abdomen cancer, and high steroid alcohol, that successively may be a leading risk issue for coronary cardiovascular disease and stroke. whereas this won't sit well with many folks, the overwhelming mass of analysis supports this. i like to recommend going feeder.

6. Eat fruits & veggies. this can be obvious, however it's superb however few veggies the general public eat. consumption fruits and veggies reduces your risk of many leading diseases, and it's one amongst the best habits to create. Eat a dish (without serious dressings, bacon or alternative meats, croutons or cheese), add green groceriess to soups or veggie chili, cook up veggies as a healthy entremots with dinner or lunch. Eat fruits with breakfast and as snacks.

7. scale back salt, and saturated/trans fats. Salt and saturated or trans fats are in numerous processed or ready foods, and that they increase risks of high pressure and high steroid alcohol, that increase risk for cardiovascular disease and stroke. Despite what the photographer worth

Foundation and others on the web tell you, saturated fat isn't healthy — browse the sources. Note that this isn't an argument within the health profession, however the "harmlessness" of saturated fats is perpetuated by the diary and meat industries, and lay writers like metropolis Taube. Cook your own healthy meals rather than consumption out or eating ready foods.

8. scale back stress. Stress may be a risk issue for cardiovascular disease and high pressure, that is itself a risk issue for stroke. change your workday in order that you're not excessively stressed, and exercise to alleviate stress.

Here's a way to amendment these habits:
Change only 1 habit at a time. It doesn't matter that habit you select. simply select one. You'll need to try to to quite one, but don't.
Create positive habits you relish. browse the last word once more — if you relish it, the habit amendment are going to be straightforward. Replace smoking with positive habits you relish that fulfill the wants that smoking currently fulfills (stress reduction, social lubrication, tedium relief, etc.). Replace red meats with healthy foods you relish.

Start as tiny as attainable. simply do five minutes the primary week, and take a look at to be consistent as attainable. Then do ten minutes. chickenfeed is far and away the foremost effective methodology I've used for dynamical habits. Slow amendment lasts.

Make it social. realize a partner or cluster to vary the habit with you, therefore you're a lot of doubtless to stay with it.

These work. I've done them over and over, and each time I follow these principles, I've modified a habit.

Healthy living isn't not possible, or maybe particularly troublesome. It's simply slower to return by than the general public look after.

Healthy habits can avoid diseases

One of the most effective ways that to keep up your health is by taking care of yourself. If you would like to measure a healthy life style and revel in your maturity while not being injected with many totally different forms of shots, then amendment your daily life style as a result of even the best very little healthy modification will cause nice edges.

Though it's troublesome to place health and fitness as a prime priority during this routine day and age, it's best to begin with baby steps can sure peak your health enormously.

Healthy Habit to Avoid unwellness # 1: Wash your hands usually

Not laundry hands before a meal is one amongst the quickest means you'll fall sick. throughout our daily chores, we tend to tend to the touch many things at a time knowing and inadvertently. because of this daily mechanism, germs will get simply transported from our hands to our mouth. Hence, continually instill the habit of laundry hands often to stay health issues at a hands distance.

Healthy Habit to Avoid unwellness # 2: Stop nose choosing

This habit of dig gold' is one amongst the worst health habits. choosing your nose perpetually will cause and unfold varied infections like cold and influenza since cold virus is passed into your body through the secretion. once touching many things then taking constant finger into your nose, can make sure that you land at the doctor's clinic. Hence, stop this awkward habit of onanism sticky substance from your nose.

Healthy Habit to Avoid unwellness # 3: Stretching is vital

Make stretching an area of your daily activities. Since we tend to pay most of our time ina workplace and infront of the pc, our muscles tend to become stiff and contracted . This stiffness will increase the chance of injuries and sever pains. To avoid these injuries, ensure to often pratice stretching each morning.

Healthy Habit to Avoid unwellness # 4: Breathe the proper means

we should always breathe from our diaphragm rather than respiratory from our chest. this alteration within the respiratory pattern will facilitate to maximise the element intake and can conjointly make sure that you keep calm. amendment your respiratory vogue to enhance the means your body functions and blood circulation.

Healthy Habit to Avoid unwellness # 5:Eat a healthy breakfast

Always ensure that you simply eat a healthy breakfast each morning. Breakfast is that the most vital meal of the day and a consumption a healthy breakfast within the morning can assist you to avoid snacking throughout the remainder of the day. Result? you'll stop upset stomach that is caused because of digestion downside and weight gain.

Healthy Habit to Avoid unwellness # 6: Bathing is sweet
Make sure you cleanse yourself totally with an honest refreshing shower gel or soap. an honest shower is critical to get rid of dirt and odor from your body and bathing conjointly helps you to revitalize. build your shower time a spoil time, by improvement every a part of your body totally to stop infection and foul odor.

Healthy Habit to Avoid unwellness # 7: Cut your nails often
Long nails won't solely build acting your daily tasks troublesome however it may also act as a bunch for infections and germs. after you bit many things, there's a large possibilities of the germs obtaining stuck into your nails – says Dr. Sunesara. These germs will pass to your mouth, after you nibble your food.

Healthy Habit to Avoid unwellness # 8: Avoid sharing personal things
Sharing personal things like razors, toothbrush and nail clips etc. will cause germ transfer. Keep your personal things only for you. ne'er share any item even together with your relations.

Healthy Habit to Avoid unwellness # 9: continually apply sunblock

Make a habit of applying an honest sunblock on your skin, whenever you venture out.This habit can keep varied skin issues like carcinoma and malignant melanoma cornered. Besides, it'll conjointly decrease skin harm and provides you a younger wanting skin for a protracted time.

Healthy Habit to Avoid unwellness # 10: Say no to sweet things

Sugary things are as toxicant as alcohol and cigarettes. Excess presence of sugar in your body, will have sever negative effects on your weight and skin. Avoid sweet things and sweet sodas to stay polygenic disease and alternative chronic diseases cornered.

Healthy Habit to Avoid unwellness # 11: Sweat it out

Give a break to your inactive life by adding a touch exercise to that. exertion often for half-hour have endless edges because it helps to keep up healthy weight, decreases tension and boosts your energy levels and mood. begin exertion keep healthy and to avoid varied vas diseases.

Healthy Habit to Avoid unwellness # 12: sensible sleep

Never compromise on your sleeping hours. an honest night's sleep for eight hours is incredibly vital to stop varied sleep disorders. Thus, continually maintain a correct schedule and proper sleeping pattern. select a snug bed and ne'er eat a significant meal late in the dead of night.

Healthy Habit to Avoid unwellness # 13: Stop worrying

The best factor favour you'll do to yourself is by avoiding stress like plague. Stress is that the reason behind varied health issues like depression, sleep disorder and heart disorder. Dr. Sunesara says – whenever stressed, apply respiratory exercise and relax yourself.

Healthy Habit to Avoid unwellness # 14: Monitor your monitor time

Reduce your monitor time, to avoid negative impact on your eyes and psychological state – says Dr. Sunesara. If your work depends on the usage of monitors then shield yourself by victimization sensible try of eye protection glasses and regulate the means you sit. Besides, ensure you avoid watching any reasonably a monitor before bed time to urge an honest nights sleep.

Healthy Habit to Avoid unwellness # 15: Drink millions of water

Drink a minimum of 8-10 glasses of water a day, betting on your physical activity. sufficient intake of water is incredibly essential to flush out toxins from your body and to rejuvenate your cells. If you are doing not drink enough water, you'll finish dehydrated yourself and therefore, exhausted.

Healthy Habit to Avoid unwellness # 16: Say no to food

Fast food is made in trans fat, sugar, spices and artificial preservatives. perpetually intense food can expand your area and cause serious health issues within the long haul like high steroid alcohol, polygenic disease and heart issues. Since sustenance is made in unhealthy fat, it raises the unhealthy steroid alcohol within the body and results in the hardening of the arteries, which might more cause plaque deposits. Hence, switch to a healthier diet and shield yourself from weight gain and alternative serious successfulness issues.

Healthy Habit to Avoid unwellness # 17: Quit smoking

Smoking even one coffin nail on a daily basis, will cause blood clots, {which may|which will} stop swift flow of the blood and therefore can cause plaque to develop in your arteries and blood vessels. Besides, you'll conjointly harm the lifetime of the nonsmoker WHO lives with you.

Healthy Habit to Avoid unwellness # 18: keep safe whereas having sex

Sex may be a enjoyable act and if you act foolish you'll land in serious health issues. continually use a prophylactic device whereas having sex to stop sexually transmitted diseases and avoid unwanted physiological state. Besides, don't be a Casanova, follow one partner for your sexual pleasures.

Healthy Habit to Avoid unwellness # 19: Respect your body and yourself

Your body is your host, learn to respect it. settle for each flaw and weaknes and learn to measure with it. If you would like to remain pleased with physiological condition and high confidence then love your body the means it's.

Healthy Habit to Avoid unwellness # 20: begin enamored vegetables

The first habit to feature in your consumption collection is to add every type of vegetables in your diet. The health edges of consumption vegetables are varied. Vegetables are loaded with fiber, essential vitamins and varied nutrients that promote physiological condition in each means.

A habit is outlined within the Merriam-Webster wordbook as a "usual means of behaving: one thing that someone will usually in a very regular and perennial way." The key word during this definition is "repeated".

Indeed, no matter activities you are doing to keep up your health, it's solely through repetition that you simply can deliver the goods your goals. Running a half-marathon once a year can at the best offer you with a lift of endorphins or at the worst, an injury. On the opposite hand, half-hour of walking or cardiopulmonary exercise many times per week, year-round, can do miracles for your quality of life and health.

Here are twenty healthy daily habits which will assist you improve your physical and mental well-being. Ideally, decide one then wait till it's totally integrated into your daily routine before choosing another!

Walking
Whenever you'll. to travel to the foodstuff or the workplace, to urge some recent air throughout your lunch break or to

visit whereas in a very new town. Walk. The minimum range of steps you must be taking a day is ten,000. it would seem to be tons, however each minute counts and gets you nearer to your goal. think about it as a game!

Stand up on an everyday basis

Prolonged inactivity may be a downside that's as current as a general lack of exercise. Staying sitting throughout hours at a time compromises the body's ability to consume fats and sugars, which might cause many health issues. Thankfully, there's a straightforward solution: get up as usually as attainable. Head to your colleague's workplace, get up once you're on the phone, or use the steps. each reason may be a sensible one to urge active every day!

Play outside

Getting some recent air a day is one amongst the best and most pleasant ways that of rising your health. Recent studies have even shown the numerous health edges of natural daylight. [1] what is more, disbursement time outside may be a great way to manage your stress. [2]

Straighten your posture

You should set regular reminders (alarms or notes) to straighten your posture! Bring your neck and hips into a neutral position, then pull your shoulder blades back and stick your chest out. an honest posture helps each muscle add AN best means and reduces pressure on your joints. within the long haul, you'll scale back your risk of obtaining back aches and within the short run, you'll feel a lot of assured, energized, and you'll be able to breathe higher.

Use your muscles

Whether to counter muscle loss related to aging, to stop osteoporosis or back aches, or to easily build any activity easier, it's in your best interest to use your muscles as usually as attainable. Take the steps, prolong a hike, do some push ups, check in for a yoga category. These are solely a number of ways that of exertion your muscles a day.

Stretch

You don't need to stretch for AN hour, you'll merely improve your flexibility by moving your body in numerous ways that a number of minutes a day. By adding a number of stretches to your daily routine, you'll increase your joint flexibility, which can scale back your risk of injury. Moreover, you'll get an immediate boost of energy because of the inflow of ventilated blood sent to your muscles and brain.

Move together with your friends
This is a two-in-one: it's fun and motivating! indeed, motivating others is one amongst the best ways that to stay yourself impelled. And by exertion together with your friends, you'll associate being active with fun and you'll need to try to to it regularly!

CHAPTER 9:

Food

Eat in sensible company

Set your screens aside and pay your time connecting with real humans. Not solely may be a voice communication a good thanks to reinforce your social bonds, it'll cause you to eat a lot of slowly. You'll set your fork down after you feel full, however not too full.

Fill half of your plate with fruits and vegetables

Many people understand this tip, however few people follow it. after you arrange your menu, add millions of salads, stews, soups, raw vegetables, gratins, purees, sautés, recent fruit, smoothies, and compotes. Fruits and veggies are jam-choked with nutrients, low in calories, and cheap. the best ingredients to a healthy diet!

Pay attention to after you feel hungry and full

How much do you have to eat each day? the solution to the current question will vary greatly and depends on your weight, gender, age, and physical activity level. That being aforesaid, an honest thanks to guarantee you're consumption enough is to listen to your hunger signals. once your abdomen growls, eat. after you feel full, stop. even though your plate isn't empty. even though somebody offers you second helpings.

Add selection to your diet
By adding selection to your menu, you'll make sure you have gotten a variety of distinctive edges from a large choice of ingredients. for example, rather than your regular morning toast, strive AN nightlong oatmeal or add otherwise colored vegetables to your cart.

Breakfast > lunch > dinner
Because you wish to focus and keep energized throughout the daytime, you must eat a filling breakfast, a medium-sized lunch, and a lightweight dinner. You'll visit bed feeling lighter and you'll get up feeling peckish. that is what you wish to begin everywhere again!

Drink lots of water

Water is crucial for staying hydrous and avoiding headaches, fatigue, and issues focusing. Keep a reusable bottle to be had and continually place it seeable to cue you to drink often. Tea, herbal tea, and nonsweet occasional are sensible choices.

Pack your lunch

Preparing your own lunch and snacks for the workplace, school, or travels may be a great way to eat the go. Not solely can you save cash, you'll avoid excess metal, sugar, fat, and chemical preservatives in meals at sustenance restaurants.

Take the time to cook

By cooking, we tend to mean taking your time throughout the week to arrange a number of easy, tasty dishes that may prevent time on busy days. It solely takes 2 hours to cook twelve muffins, slice a melon and vegetables, marinade bean curd, and cook quinoa.

Putting away your smartphone may appear like a huge challenge. however being connected 24/7 will have negative facet effects on your memory, creativity, and productivity. Disconnect a minimum of one hour a day and provides your brain a well-deserved break!

Breathe

Take your time to require deep breaths. With everything that's happening around you, you may solely be taking short, shallow breaths. disbursement a number of moments respiratory deeply will calm your mind and supply physical edges, like lowering your pressure and rate. It may also assist you manage your stress.

Enjoy a micro-vacation

Every day? If you can! It solely takes half AN hour. A micro-vacation merely suggests that an instant in your day after you will rest and relax. Lie back and stare off into the gap.

Let your brain wander. You'll be shocked at however helpful this may be for your creative thinking and energy levels!

Sleep

Sleep, a bit like exercise and a healthy diet, is one amongst the pillars of excellent health. obtaining enough sleep (between seven and eight hours each night) on an everyday basis can have a positive impact on your mood, memory, longevity, also as your psychological feature and physical performance.

Smile

This is a straightforward habit to adopt and can greatly impact your mood. merely raising the corners of your mouth produces endorphins, providing instant happiness!

In conclusion, one amongst the benefits of adopting healthy life style habits is that it's attainable to keep up them forever. This isn't always attainable with extreme solutions that usually turn out to be a furor. By that specialize in healthy life style habits, you'll guarantee your success is long-lasting!

Morning Habits That assist you change state

No matter what your weight loss goals are, losing weight will feel not possible sometimes.

However, shedding a number of pounds doesn't need to involve an entire overhaul of your current diet and life style. In fact, creating a number of tiny changes to your morning routine will assist you change state and keep it off.

1. Eat a High-Protein Breakfast

There's an honest reason breakfast is taken into account the foremost vital meal of the day.

What you eat for breakfast will set the course for your entire day. It determines if you'll feel full and glad till lunch, or if you'll be heading to the coin machine before your mid-morning snack.

Eating a high-protein breakfast might facilitate cut cravings and aid in weight loss.

In one study in twenty adolescent women, consumption a high-protein breakfast reduced post-meal cravings a lot of effectively than a normal-protein breakfast.

Another tiny study showed that consumption a high-protein breakfast was related to less fat gain and reduced daily intake and hunger, compared to a normal-protein breakfast.

Protein may additionally aid weight loss by decreasing levels of hormone, the "hunger hormone" that's answerable for increasing craving.

In fact, one study in fifteen men found that a high-protein breakfast suppressed hormone secretion a lot of effectively than a high-carb breakfast.

To help get your break day to an honest begin, think about supermolecule sources like eggs, Greek yoghourt, pot cheese, loco and chia seeds.

Studies show that a high-protein breakfast might aid weight loss by reducing cravings, craving and hormone secretion.

2. Drink lots of Water

Starting your morning with a glass or 2 of water is a straightforward thanks to enhance weight loss.

Water will facilitate increase your energy expenditure, or the amount of calories your body burns, for a minimum of hour.

In one tiny study, drinking sixteen.9 fluid ounces (500 ml) of water diode to a 30% increase in rate, on the average.

Another study found that overweight ladies WHO increased their water intake to over thirty four ounces (one liter) per day lost an additional 4.4 pounds (2 kg) over one year, while not creating the other changes in their diet or exercise routine.

What's a lot of, potable might scale back craving and food intake in some people.

One study in twenty four older adults showed that drinking sixteen.9 fluid ounces (500 ml) of water reduced the amount of calories consumed at breakfast by 13%.

In fact, most studies on the subject have shown that drinking 34-68 ounces (1-2 liters) of water per day will aid in weight loss.

Starting your morning with water and staying well hydrous throughout the day may be a good way to spice up weight loss with stripped-down effort.

Increasing your water intake has been related to a rise in weight loss and energy expenditure, also as a decrease in craving and food intake.

3. Weigh Yourself

Stepping on the dimensions and deliberation yourself every morning is an efficient methodology to extend motivation and improve self-control.

Several studies have associated deliberation yourself daily with bigger weight loss.

For instance, a study in forty seven individuals found that those that weighed themselves daily lost concerning thirteen pounds (6 kg) a lot of over six months than those who weighed themselves less usually.

Another study reportable that adults WHO weighed themselves daily lost a mean of nine.7 pounds (4.4 kg) over a biennial amount, whereas those that weighed themselves once a month gained four.6 pounds (2.1 kg).

Weighing yourself each morning may also facilitate foster healthy habits and behaviors that will promote weight loss.

In one massive study, frequent self-weighing was related to improved restraint. what is more, those that stopped deliberation themselves often were a lot of doubtless to report increased calorie intake and decreased self-discipline.

For best results, weigh yourself right after you get up. Do therefore once victimization the lavatory and before you eat or drink something.

Additionally, bear in mind that your weight may fluctuate daily and may be influenced by a range of things. specialize in the massive image and appearance for overall weight loss trends, instead of obtaining fixated on tiny daily changes.

Studies have found that daily self-weighing is also related to a lot of weight loss and increased restraint.

4. Get Some Sun

Opening the curtains to let in some daylight or disbursement a number of further minutes outside every morning will facilitate kickstart your weight loss.

One tiny study found that exposure to even moderate levels of sunshine at sure times of the day will have an influence on weight.

Moreover, AN animal study found that exposure to actinic ray helped suppress weight gain in mice fed a high-fat diet.

Exposure to daylight is additionally the most effective thanks to meet your ergocalciferol wants. Some studies have found that meeting your ergocalciferol necessities will aid in weight loss and even stop weight gain.

In one study, 218 overweight and rotund ladies took either ergocalciferol supplements or a placebo for one year. At the top of the study, those that met their ergocalciferol demand lost a mean of seven pounds (3.2 kg) quite those with inadequate ergocalciferol blood levels.

Another study followed four,659 older ladies for four years and located that higher levels of ergocalciferol were joined to less weight gain.

The amount of sun exposure you wish will vary supported your skin kind, the season and your location. However, holding in some daylight or sitting outside for 10–15 minutes every morning might have a helpful impact on weight loss.

Sun exposure might have AN influence on weight. daylight may also assist you meet your ergocalciferol wants, which can facilitate increase weight loss and forestall weight gain.

5. apply attentiveness

Mindfulness may be a apply that involves totally that specialize in the current moment and transferral awareness to your thoughts and feelings.

The apply has been shown to boost weight loss and promote healthy consumption habits.

For example, AN analysis of nineteen studies found that mindfulness-based interventions increased weight loss and reduced obesity-related consumption behaviors.

Another review had similar findings, noting that attentiveness coaching resulted in vital weight loss in 68% of the studies reviewed.

Practicing attentiveness is straightforward. to urge started, strive disbursement 5 minutes every morning sitting well in a very calm area and connecting together with your senses.

Some studies have found that attentiveness will increase weight loss and promote healthy consumption behaviors.

6. Squeeze in Some Exercise

Getting in some physical activity very first thing within the morning will facilitate boost weight loss.

One study in fifty overweight ladies measured the results of cardiopulmonary exercise at totally different times of the day.

While there wasn't a lot of distinction noted in specific food cravings between those that exercised within the morning versus the afternoon, figuring out within the morning was related to the next level of satiation.

Exercising within the morning may additionally facilitate keep blood glucose levels steady throughout the day. Low blood glucose may end up in several negative symptoms, as well as excessive hunger.

One study in thirty five individuals with kind one polygenic disease showed that figuring out within the morning was related to improved blood glucose management.

However, these studies targeted on terribly specific populations ANd show an association, instead of deed. a lot of analysis on the results of morning exercise within the general population is required.

Some studies have found that exertion within the morning is also related to increased satiation and improved blood glucose management.

7. Pack Your Lunch

Making the trouble to arrange and pack your lunch prior time is a straightforward thanks to build higher food decisions and increase weight loss.

A large study as well as forty,554 individuals found that meal coming up with was related to higher diet quality, a lot of diet selection and a lower risk of fleshiness.

Another study found that consumption home-cooked meals a lot of often was related to improved diet quality and a decreased risk of excess body fat.

In fact, those that Ate home-cooked meals a minimum of 5 times per week were 28% less doubtless to be overweight than those who solely ate home-cooked meals 3 times or less per week.

Try setting aside a number of hours one night per week to arrange and prepare your meals in order that within the morning you'll simply grab your lunch and go.

Studies show that meal coming up with and consumption home-cooked meals are related to improved diet quality and a lower risk of fleshiness.

8. Sleep Longer

Going to bed a touch earlier or setting your timer later to squeeze in some further sleep might facilitate increase weight loss.

Several studies have found that sleep deprivation is also related to AN increased craving.

One tiny study found that sleep restriction increased hunger and cravings, particularly for high-carb, high-calorie foods.

Lack of sleep has conjointly been joined to a rise in calorie intake.

In one study, twelve participants consumed a mean of 559 a lot of calories once obtaining simply four hours of sleep, compared to after they got a full eight hours.

Establishing a healthy sleep schedule may be a important part of weight loss, along side consumption well and exertion. to maximise your results, aim for a minimum of eight hours of sleep per night.

Studies show that sleep deprivation might increase craving and cravings, also as calorie intake.

9. Switch up Your Commute

While driving is also one amongst the foremost convenient ways that to urge to figure, it's going to not be therefore nice for your area.

Research shows that walking, biking or by using public transportation is also tied to a lower weight and reduced risk of weight gain.

One study followed 822 individuals over four years and located that those that commuted by automotive attended gain a lot of weight than non-car commuters.

Similarly, a study as well as fifteen,777 individuals showed that using public transportation or active ways of transport, like walking or biking, was related to a considerably lower body mass index and body fat proportion, compared to using non-public transportation.

Changing up your commute even a number of times per week is also a straightforward thanks to build weight loss.

Walking, biking and using public transportation have all been related to less weight gain and lower weight and body fat, compared to driving to figure.

10. begin trailing Your Intake

Keeping a food diary to trace what you eat is an efficient thanks to facilitate boost weight loss and keep yourself responsible.

One study half-tracked weight loss in 123 individuals for one year and located that finishing a food journal was related to a bigger quantity of weight loss.

Another study showed that participants who often used a trailing system to self-monitor their diet and exercise lost a lot of weight than those that failed to regularly use the tracking system.

Similarly, a study of 220 rotund ladies found that the frequent and consistent use of a self-monitoring tool helped improve long-run weight management.

Try using AN app or maybe simply a pen and paper to record what you eat and drink, beginning together with your initial meal of the day.

Studies have found that employing a food diary to trace your intake will facilitate increase weight loss.

Making a number of tiny changes to your morning habits is a straightforward and effective thanks to increase weight loss.

Practicing healthy behaviors within the morning may also get your day started on the proper foot and set you up for fulfillment.

For best results, ensure you mix these morning habits with a all-around diet and healthy life style.

Have a transparent goal. It ought to be one that anyone within the world will live and perceive.

2. Drink tea. analysis suggests that those that drink tea – black, inexperienced or white, as long as it's from real tea versus tea – have lower BMIs and fewer body fat than those that don't consume tea.

3. Eat cayenne pepper. A study printed within the British Journal of Nutrition showed that in comparison to placebo, chemical irritant – the active ingredient in cayenne – increased fat burning.

4. Decrease/eliminate processed carbs. they are doing nothing for you outside of making a favourable setting for gaining fat.

5. Eat a lot of veggies. They fill you up, while not providing several kilojoules. simply avoid the high-kilojoule dressings.

6. Eat a lot of fruit. nobody ever gained weight from consumption a lot of fruit. which includes the supposed "high sugar" fruits like bananas and melons.

7. elevate weights. serious weights. Build a lot of muscle, burn a lot of kilojoules.

8. prevent rest time between sets. this may keep your rate elevated, inflicting a rise in kilojoules burned.

9. Do intervals. Study once study after study continues to indicate intervals are more practical and time economical than longer activity performed at a lower intensity.

10. Eat a lot of supermolecule. commutation refined carbohydrates with lean supermolecule won't solely facilitate satiate you, however also will increase your metabolism – through one thing referred to as the thermal impact of food.

11. Eat supermolecule a lot of often. It's vital to conjointly time your intake so you're consumption supermolecule often throughout the day – not simply in one payment, like most do at dinner. each meal and snack ought to embrace some supermolecule.

12. Supplement with animal oil. A study printed in Lipids fed mice diets increased epa and DHA – a.k.a. fish oil. The researchers learnt that the mice fed diets higher in polyunsaturated fatty acid fats had considerably less accumulation of body fat. alternative studies have shown similar results.

13. Do full body exercises. Think: Squats, deadlifts, chin-ups and pushups. You'll get a lot of bang for your buck out of every exertion.

14. Cycle your carb intake supported your activity level. Sure, carbs are vital. however on the times you don't calculate, you merely don't would like as several compared to the times you exercise exhausting. Rule of thumb: The a lot of active you're, the a lot of carbs you'll eat, and the other way around.

15. begin your meals with a dish. dish can offer some bulk to assist fill you up – in order that you eat less kilojoules overall.

16. Don't forget the fibre. think about fibre sort of a sponge; it absorbs water and causes you to feel full.

17. Drink water. prof Dr Brenda Davy and her team from Virginia school University found that giving individuals 2 cups of water before every meal resulted in bigger weight loss once twelve weeks. The reason? It helps fill you up.

18. Add beans to your salads. It's a pleasant thanks to add some further fibre, supermolecule and healthy carbs.

19. Replace one meal on a daily basis with an oversized dish and lean supermolecule. this can be a straightforward thanks to instantly improve your diet.

20. Keep a food journal. There's no higher thanks to track what you're putting in place your mouth.

21. Watch your parts. Avoid the buffet line and ne'er supersize. Instead ensure you're following what the nutrition label recommends for a serving.

22. Switch to kilojoule-free drinks. All kilojoules count, whether or not they're liquid or solid. therefore unless it's milk, elect tea or water. Or one thing i used to be introduced to within the Netherlands – massive bunches of mint, lemon and predicament.

23. Weigh yourself. Studies show daily weigh-ins facilitate enhance weight loss efforts. Don't live and die by the amount. And, of course, a scale doesn't decipher between fat

and lean body mass, however it will still be of profit to stay things "in check".

24. Eat whole eggs. Daily. A study printed a few years past showed that those that Ate whole eggs versus a beigel for breakfast ate less at future meal. the same study showed consumption whole eggs will increase high-density lipoprotein steroid alcohol.

25. Eat breakfast. A review printed within the yankee Journal of Clinical Nutrition showed that those that eat breakfast are a lot of booming with long-run weight maintenance. alternative analysis has shown constant for weight loss. Grab hardboiled eggs, disorganised eggs, Greek food, a bit of fruit and few loco, or build a smoothie. It doesn't need to be fancy.

26. Eat the majority of your meals within the A.M. Then eat more and more less throughout the day. A study printed within the Journal of Nutrition showed that consumption most of your kilojoules earlier in the day completely influences weight changes.

27. To burn a lot of kilojoules, keep upright. this suggests not sitting before of a pc, TV, phone, etc., all day long. Stand and you'll burn a lot of and be more productive.

28. Use the steps. That's right: Skip the escalator and elevator. This won't build or break success, however each

little helps.

29. Eat low-energy, dense foods. These are foods that are high in water and lower in calories, like fruit, veggies, soups and salads. Studies at Penn State University have shown that the inclusion of those foods helps people eat less total kilojoules overall.

30. Don't grocery search hungry. If you do, you'll obtain everything within the aisle – rather than sticking out to your list. And most of the time, the foods you get once hungry can the types that sabotage your weight-loss efforts.

31. Replace facet dishes with steamed veggies. Restaurants can usually permit you to substitute the fries or chips with steamed veggies. All you've got to try to to is raise.

32. Bake, don't fry. It's pretty easy extremely. Ditch the pans and switch thereon kitchen appliance.

33. Use the fat-burner in your backyard: Your grill. And as South Africans we tend to love an honest braai. simply skip the staff of life and select a tasty dish as a facet instead.

34. Order dressing on the facet. however here's the larger secret: Dip your fork in dressing, then within the dish. this protects a lot a lot of dressing than if one was to order it on the facet, then pour the complete cup on the dish anyway. Fewer kilojoules equal less weight.

35. within the airport: Carry your bags, don't roll it. Again, not a deal breaker in terms of success – simply otherwise to extend energy expenditure.

36. Skip the "Venti lattes" and elect plain occasional. (Or higher nonetheless, tea.) Those extra-large "designer" coffees will pack a belly-inflating a pair of 000 or a lot of kilojoules per serving!

37. Embrace oats. Plain oatmeal can facilitate fill you up quite the high sugar breakfast counterparts. Moreover, one serving provides tons less kilojoules than the sugary alternatives.

38. Fidget. A study printed within the journal Science showed that those that fidgeted a lot of usually – as an example, modified their posture often – weighed but those that didn't. This further movement was termed NEAT (non-exercise activity thermogenesis).

39. Laugh usually. A study bestowed on fleshiness found those that laughed exhausting for roughly ten to fifteen minutes day by day burned a further forty to one hundred sixty kilojoules per day. Multiply that by 365 and people kilojoules will add up!

40. Leave one thing on your plate at the top of the meal. each little counts.

Read more: The four mistakes that are creating you fat

41. once bent on eat, split a meal. The parts are typically sufficiently big to feed a family.

42. Skip course. Come on, you recognize you wish to and likelihood is you aren't even hungry after you reach for that sweet treat.

43. Don't socialise round the food tables at parties. You're a lot of doubtless to munch senselessly, even supposing you'll not be hungry.

44. Don't eat your kid's leftovers. each little of food adds up, {including|as we tend toll as|together with} what we decision "BLTs" (bites, licks and tastes).

45. Keep chips, dips and alternative high fat junk foods out of the house. It's not concerning willpower; it's about being realistic.

46. If you've got a dog, take him for a walk. It's higher for each him and you than simply holding him out the rear.

Morning within the town. Young man walking together with his do

47. If you don't have a pet, provide to run a neighbour's dog. build friends; change state.

48. Use smaller plates and bowls. there'll be less space for you to extra service and it makes less food feels like a lot of.

49. Skip buffets. It's a gone conclusion: If you don't, you'll desire you've got to urge your money's price and overindulge.

50. Slow down. It takes roughly fifteen to twenty minutes for your abdomen to sense it's full. If you wolf your food sort of a starving dog, you'll doubtless out-eat your hunger.

51. Decrease your food intake by four hundred kilojoules per day. on paper this interprets to losing nearly 450g per month (450g = fourteen 600 kilojoules) – with hardly any effort.

52. obtain a measuring instrument and accumulate a minimum of ten 000 steps day by day. It feels like everyone is doing it therefore why shouldn't you too?

53. once attainable, walk or bike to try to your errands. The additional bonus? You'll save on gasoline too.

54. Don't render bulk. The a lot of that's there, the a lot of that you'll eat.

55. Plan ahead. If you fail to arrange, you propose to fail.

56. Keep thereforeme healthy snacks – like loco – in your compartment so you're ready the least bit times.

57. Take before footage. Studies have shown that those that take weight-loss progress pics lose a lot of weight than those who don't.

58. Get new friends. If your friends like dish, wings, nachos and brewage on an everyday basis, realize friends WHO are similar and need to be healthy. analysis has recommended that friends enhance (or will hurt) success.

59. place yourself initial. many folks (women in particular) place everybody else prior themselves and let their health fall by the facet.

60. Remember: It's not all or nothing. If you fall off the bandwagon, jump right back on. Don't let yourself still fall till all progress has been lost.

61. get up early to exercise. You're a lot of doubtless to urge it done if you don't wait till once work.

If weight loss may be a goal for you, then you almost certainly already know—whether or not you would like to admit it—that there's no quickie once it involves creating it happen and making it last. perhaps you've even learned that lesson the exhausting means. (Maybe quite once.) therefore ditch the furor diets and take a glance at the massive image. It's vital to recollect that losing weight isn't concerning starving yourself, which forceful measures will place a dangerous strain on your body.

The real key to finding and maintaining a healthy weight is finding and maintaining a healthy life style. Here's some healthy-living knowledge to assist guide you on your means.

Focus on food initial.
Your initial thought may well be that you simply need to hit the athletic facility to change state, however it's not enough to figure out exhausting if you're not consumption well. analysis has found that exercise alone isn't as effective for weight loss as dietary changes. after you place them along you've got a direction for long-run success.

Eat quality calories, not empty ones.
Sugar may be a drug. however you'll kick the habit. prolong a sweets hiatus—a month is right, however do what you can—and you'll see the cravings begin to diminish. Then it'll be easier to avoid sugar-laden foods that don't offer your body the nutrients it wants, leave you hungry, and cause you to placed on weight. From there you'll focus your attention on whole grains, fruits and vegetables, fish and lean supermolecule. examine these twenty superfoods that are nice for weight loss.

And eat enough calories to really sustain you.

Your body wants food, so eat it. the thought here is to make consumption habits that you simply will really stick to, not starve yourself. If you would like to use an advert diet to assist you select what you set on your plate.

Definitely don't skip breakfast.
Eating breakfast facilitates maintain stable blood glucose levels and may help keep you full all day therefore you don't snack. In fact, a study of individuals WHO with success shed weight and unbroken it off, found that just about eighty p.c Ate breakfast a day as a part of their weight-loss strategy. Leave the croissants and muffins within the pastry shop— they really cause you to hungrier later—and elect supermolecule and whole grains to begin the day. Here are ten scrumptious protein-packed breakfasts to do. What the euphemism, here are five a lot of.

Pay attention to what you eat—literally.
They say you must watch what you eat. however what we're expression is you must really watch what you eat, as you're consumption it. inspect the food, soak up the smell and therefore the texture, relish it as you chew. It's not almost about tasting, it's concerning being aware about what you're golf shot into your body. after you dine in front of the TV or

your pc, otherwise you graze all day long at the workplace, you finish up with what primarily amounts to meal memory loss.

You don't bear in mind what you ate—and you're doubtless to eat {more|additional|a heap of} (a lot more) than you meant to. strive keeping a food diary for per week or 2 to urge to bear with what you're really consumption a day and to spot patterns that may be busybodied together with your arrange. for example, if you're continually starving by suppertime and going back for seconds and thirds, perhaps you wish to schedule in a very healthy snack at four P.M. analysis finds time and once more that observation what you eat helps you change state.

Drink tons of water and not a lot of soda, juice or alcohol.
Your cells would like water to perform, therefore it's crucial to stay hydrating throughout the day. (Here are twelve straightforward ways that to drink a lot of water a day.) Yes, you'll get a number of that fluid from drinks that aren't simply plain water, however watch out that you're not gulping down loads of supernumerary calories. Soda and juice—despite its victuals content—are jam-choked with sugar. Alcohol is another supply of sneaky empty calories. If you're progressing to imbibe, strive these ten lower-calorie

cocktails.

Don't skimp on sleep.

Sleep may be a astonishingly vital think about losing weight and keeping it off. those that are sleep underprivileged eat a lot of calories throughout the day and are more doubtless to place on weight.

Find a variety of exercise that you simply really need to try to.

Combining exercise with diet has been shown to be more practical for weight loss than diet alone. You'll be a lot of doubtless to stay to an everyday program of physical activity if you truly, you know, enjoy it. would like some further motivation? Get a exertion brother. You'll be less inclined to skip a run if you recognize your friend is awaiting you within the park. Here's the thin on the most effective thanks to calculate for weight loss.

And then keep doing it.

Keeping weight off may be a constant balance,. and regular physical activity may be a huge a part of creating it last. You can't simply go extremely exhausting in the future and suppose, OK I'm sensible for a number of weeks. consumption healthy and exertion need to become a part of life. and that they will! and, physical activity is concerning quite simply burning off calories. you wish to strengthen your muscles, too. The cool factor is, muscles assign calories simply by existing, therefore it's solely progressing to assist you within the long haul to strengthen.

Pick up any diet book and it'll claim to carry all the answers to with success losing all the burden you want—and keeping it off. Some claim the secret's to eat less and exercise additional, others that low fat is that the solely thanks to go, whereas others order extirpation carbs. So, what must you believe?

The truth is there's no "one size fits all" answer to permanent healthy weight loss. What works for one person might not work for you, since our bodies respond otherwise to completely different foods, counting on genetic science and different health factors. to search out the strategy of weight loss that's right for you'll possible take time and need patience, commitment, and a few experimentation with completely different foods and diets.

While some folks respond well to reckoning calories or similar restrictive ways, others respond higher to having additional freedom in designing their weight-loss programs. Being absolve to merely avoid cooked foods or decrease on refined carbs will set them up for achievement.

So, don't get too discouraged if a diet that worked for someone else doesn't work for you. And don't beat yourself up if a diet proves too restrictive for you to stay with. Ultimately, a diet is merely right for you if it's one you'll be able to continue over time.

Remember: whereas there's no simple fix to losing weight, there are lots of steps you'll be able to go for develop a healthier relationship with food, curb emotional triggers to gula, and succeed a healthy weight.

Four widespread weight loss ways

1. Cut calories

Some specialists believe that with success managing your weight comes all the way down to a straightforward equation: If you eat fewer calories than you burn, you melt off. Sounds simple, right? Then why is losing weight therefore hard?

Weight loss isn't a linear event over time. once you cut calories, you will drop weight for the primary few weeks, for instance, so one thing changes. You eat identical variety of calories however you lose less weight or no weight in the least. That's as a result of once you melt off you're losing water and lean tissue moreover as fat, your metabolism slows, and your body changes in different ways in which. So, so as to continue dropping weight every week, you wish to continue cutting calories.

A calorie isn't perpetually a calorie. ingestion one hundred calories of high laevulose syrup, for instance, will have a special impact on your body than ingestion one hundred calories of broccoli. The trick for sustained weight loss is to ditch the foods that are jam-choked with calories however don't cause you to feel full (like candy) and replace them with foods that fill you up while not being loaded with calories (like vegetables).

Many people don't perpetually eat merely to satisfy hunger. we have a tendency to conjointly communicate food for comfort or to alleviate stress—which will quickly derail any weight loss arrange.

2. Cut carbs

A different means of viewing weight loss identifies the matter as not one among overwhelming too several calories, however rather the means the body accumulates fat when overwhelming carbohydrates—in explicit the role of the secretion hormone. once you eat a meal, carbohydrates from the food enter your blood as aldohexose. so as to stay your glucose levels under control, your body perpetually burns off this aldohexose before it burns off fat from a meal.

If you eat a carbohydrate-rich meal (lots of food, rice, bread, or fries, for instance), your body releases hormone to assist with the inflow of all this aldohexose into your blood. moreover as control glucose levels, hormone will 2 things: It prevents your fat cells from emotional fat for the body to burn as fuel (because its priority is to burn off the glucose) and it creates additional fat cells for storing everything that your body can't burn off. The result's that you just gain weight and your body currently needs additional fuel to burn, therefore you eat additional. Since hormone solely burns carbohydrates, you crave carbs so begins a positive feedback of overwhelming carbs and gaining weight. To melt off, the reasoning goes, you wish to interrupt this cycle by reducing carbs.

Most low-carb diets advocate commutation carbs with supermolecule and fat, that may have some negative semipermanent effects on your health. If you are doing attempt a low-carb diet, you'll be able to cut back your risks and limit your intake of saturated and trans fats by selecting lean meats, fish and eater sources of protein, low-fat farm merchandise, and ingestion lots of unifoliate inexperienced and non-starchy vegetables.

3. Cut fat

It's a mainstay of the many diets: if you don't wish to induce fat, don't eat fat. Walk down any food market aisle and you'll be bombarded with reduced-fat snacks, dairy, and packaged meals. however whereas our low-fat choices have exploded, therefore have blubber rates. So, why haven't low-fat diets worked for additional of us?

Not all fat is unhealthy. Healthy or "good" fats will really facilitate to regulate your weight, moreover as manage your moods and fight fatigue. Unsaturated fats found in avocados, nuts, seeds, soy milk, tofu, and fatty fish will facilitate fill you up, whereas adding a bit tasty oil to a plate of vegetables, for instance, will build it easier to eat healthy food and improve the general quality of your diet.

We often build the incorrect trade-offs. several people build the error of swapping fat for the empty calories of sugar and refined carbohydrates. rather than ingestion whole-fat dairy product, for example, we have a tendency to eat low- or no-fat versions that are jam-choked with sugar to create up for the loss of style. Or we have a tendency to swap our fatty breakfast bacon for a gem or doughnut that causes fast spikes in glucose.

4. Follow the Mediterranean diet

The Mediterranean diet emphasizes ingestion sensible fats and good carbs along side massive quantities of contemporary fruits and vegetables, nuts, fish, and olive oil —and solely modest amounts of meat and cheese. The Mediterranean diet is over with reference to food, though. Regular physical activity and sharing meals with others are major elements.

Whatever weight loss strategy you are attempting, it's vital to remain actuated and avoid common fasting pitfalls, like emotional ingestion.

Control emotional ingestion

We don't perpetually eat merely to satisfy hunger. only too usually, we have a tendency to communicate food once we're stressed or anxious, which may wreck any diet and put on the pounds. does one eat once you're troubled, bored, or lonely? does one snack ahead of the TV at the tip of a disagreeable day? Recognizing your emotional ingestion triggers will build all the distinction in your weight-loss efforts. If you eat once you're:

Stressed – notice healthier ways in which to calm yourself. Try yoga, meditation, or soaking during a hot bathtub.

Low on energy – notice different mid-afternoon pick-me-ups. attempt walking round the block, paying attention to energizing music, or taking a brief nap.

Lonely or bored – reach resolute others rather than reaching for the icebox. decision a follower who causes you to laugh, take your dog for a walk, or visit the library, mall, or park—anywhere there's folks.

Practice aware ingestion instead
Avoid distractions whereas ingestion. attempt to not eat whereas operating, observance TV, or driving. It's too simple to senselessly scarf out.
Pay attention. Eat slowly, feeding the smells and textures of your food. If your mind wanders, gently come your attention to your food and the way it tastes.
Mix things up to specialise in the expertise of ingestion. attempt using chopsticks instead of a fork, or use your utensils together with your non-dominant hand.
Stop ingestion before you're full. It takes time for the signal to succeed in your brain that you've had enough. Don't feel indebted to perpetually clean your plate.

Stay actuated
Permanent weight loss needs creating healthy changes to your way and food selections. to remain motivated:
Find a cheering section. Social support means that tons. Programs like Jenny Craig and Weight Watchers use cluster

support to impact weight loss and long healthy ingestion. hunt down support—whether within the variety of family, friends, or a support group—to get the encouragement you wish.

Slow and steady wins the race. Losing weight too quick will take a toll on your mind and body, creating you are feeling sluggish, drained, and sick. Aim to lose one to 2 pounds every week therefore you're losing fat instead of water and muscle.

Set goals to stay you actuated. short-run goals, like desperate to work into a swimsuit for the summer, typically don't work moreover as desperate to feel more assured or become healthier for your children's sakes. once temptation strikes, specialise in the advantages you'll reap from being healthier.

Use tools to trace your progress. Smartphone apps, fitness trackers, or just keeping a journal will assist you keep track of the food you eat, the calories you burn, and also the weight you lose. Seeing the ends up in black and white will assist you keep actuated.

Get lots of sleep. Lack of sleep stimulates your craving therefore you would like additional food than normal; at identical time, it stops you feeling happy, creating you would like to stay ingestion. Sleep deprivation can even have an effect on your motivation, therefore aim for eight hours of quality sleep an evening.

Cut down on sugar and refined carbs
Whether or not you're specifically planning to cut carbs, most people consume unhealthy amounts of sugar and refined carbohydrates like bread, dish dough, pasta, pastries, white flour, white rice, and sweet breakfast cereals. commutation refined carbs with their whole-grain counterparts and eliminating candy and desserts is merely a part of the answer, though. Sugar is hidden in foods as various as canned soups and vegetables, spaghetti sauce, margarine, and plenty of reduced fat foods. Since your body gets all it wants from sugar present in food, all this superimposed sugar amounts to nada however tons of empty calories and unhealthy spikes in your blood sugar.

Less sugar will mean a slimmer waist
Calories obtained from laevulose (found in candied beverages like soda and processed foods like doughnuts, muffins, and candy) are additional possible to feature to fat around your belly. cutting short on candied foods will mean a slimmer waist moreover as a lower risk of polygenic disease.

Fill up with fruit, veggies, and fiber

Even if you're cutting calories, that doesn't essentially mean you've got to eat less food. High-fiber foods like fruit, vegetables, beans, and whole grains are higher in volume and take longer to digest, creating them filling—and nice for weight-loss.

It's usually okay to eat the maximum amount contemporary fruit and non-starchy vegetables as you want—you'll feel full before you've overdone it on the calories.

Eat vegetables raw or steamed, not cooked or breaded, and dress them with herbs and spices or a bit oil for flavor.

Add fruit to low sugar cereal—blueberries, strawberries, sliced bananas. You'll still get pleasure from voluminous sweetness, however with fewer calories, less sugar, and additional fiber.

Bulk out sandwiches by adding healthy produce selections like lettuce, tomatoes, sprouts, cucumbers, and avocado.

Snack on carrots or celery with hoummos rather than a high-calorie chips and dip.

Add additional veggies to your favorite main courses to create your dish more substantial. Even food and stir-fries will be diet-friendly if you utilize less noodles and additional vegetables.

Start your meal with dish or {vegetable thereforeup|petite marmite|minestrone|soup} to assist fill you up so you eat less of your entrée.

CHAPTER 10:

Take charge of your food setting

Set yourself up for weight-loss success by taking charge of your food environment: once you eat, what proportion you eat, and what foods you create simply on the market.

Cook your own meals reception. this permits you to regulate each portion size and what goes in to the food. building and packaged foods usually contain tons additional sugar, unhealthy fat, and calories than food parched at home—plus the portion sizes tend to be larger.

Serve yourself smaller parts. Use little plates, bowls, and cups to create your parts seem larger. Don't eat of huge bowls or directly from food containers, that makes it tough to assess what proportion you've ingested.

Eat early. Studies counsel that overwhelming additional of your daily calories at breakfast and fewer at dinner will assist you drop more pounds. ingestion a bigger, healthy breakfast will jump begin your metabolism, stop you feeling hungry throughout the day, and provides you longer to burn off the calories.

Fast for fourteen hours every day. attempt to eat dinner earlier within the day so quick till breakfast following morning. ingestion only if you're most active and giving your digestion an extended break could aid weight loss.

Plan your meals and snacks prior time. you'll be able to produce your own little portion snacks in plastic luggage or containers. ingestion on a schedule can assist you avoid eating once you aren't really hungry.

Drink additional water. Thirst will usually be confused with hunger, therefore by potable you'll be able to avoid additional calories.

Limit the quantity of tempting foods you've got reception. If you share a room with non-dieters, store indulgent foods out of sight.

Get moving

The degree to that exercise aids weight loss is receptive discussion, however the advantages go means on the far side burning calories. Exercise can increase your metabolism and improve your outlook—and it's one thing you'll be able to like right away. opt for a walk, stretch, move around and you'll have additional energy and motivation to tackle the opposite steps in your weight-loss program.

Lack time for an extended elbow grease? 3 10-minute spurts of exercise per day will be even as sensible jointly 30-minute workout.

Remember: something is best than nothing. take off slowly with little amounts of physical activity day after day. Then, as you begin to melt off and have additional energy, you'll notice it easier to become additional physically active.

Find exercise you get pleasure from. attempt walking with a follower, dancing, hiking, cycling, taking part in Frisbee with a dog, enjoying a pickup game of basketball, or taking part in activity-based video games together with your children.

Keeping the burden Off

You may have detected the wide quoted data point that 95% of individuals who melt off on a diet can regain it inside a couple of years—or even months. whereas there isn't abundant exhausting proof to support that claim, it's true that a lot of weight-loss plans fail within the future. usually that's just because diets that are too restrictive are terribly exhausting to keep up over time. However, that doesn't mean your weight loss makes an attempt are doomed to failure. aloof from it.

Since it had been established in 1994, The National Weight management written account (NWCR) within the u. s., has half-tracked over ten,000 people who have lost vital amounts of weight and unbroken it off for long periods of your time. The study has found that participants who've been thriving in maintaining their weight loss share some common ways. no matter diet you utilize to melt off within the initial place, adopting these habits could assist you to stay it off:

Stay physically active. thriving dieters within the study exercise for regarding hour, usually walking.

Keep a food log. Recording what you eat a day helps to stay you responsible and actuated.

Eat breakfast a day. most ordinarily within the study, it's cereal and fruit. ingestion breakfast boosts metabolism and staves off hunger later within the day.

Eat additional fiber and fewer unhealthy fat than the standard yank diet.

Regularly check the size. deliberation yourself weekly could assist you to notice any little gains in weight, sanctionative you to promptly take corrective action before the matter escalates.

Watch less tv. cutting short on the time spent sitting ahead of a screen will be a key a part of adopting a additional active way and preventing weight gain.

Conclusion

Emotional eating is when individuals use diet as a way of dealing with emotions, rather than fulfilling hunger. We've all been there, stopping out of frustration or downing cookie after cookie with a whole bag of chips while cramming for a big test. But emotional eating may affect weight, safety, and overall well-being when done a lot. But now you have all the information needed inside this books to overcome all the difficulties along you journey to be free!

CPSIA information can be obtained
at www.ICGtesting.com
Printed in the USA
LVHW050602290121
677803LV00008B/210

9 781801 381307